D0712754

Rational Diagnosis and Treatment

Fourth Edition

Rational Diagnosis and Treatment

Evidence-Based Clinical Decision-Making
Fourth Edition

Peter C. Gøtzsche
Consultant Physician, Director of The Nordic Cochrane Centre
Rigshospitalet, Copenhagen, Denmark

BICENTENNIAL
1807
WILEY
2007
BICENTENNIAL

John Wiley & Sons, Ltd

First published (HR Wulff) 1976
Second edition 1981
Third edition (HR Wulff and PC Gøtzsche) 2000

(Previous editions Blackwell)

Also published in: Danish (1973, 1981, 1987, 1997, 2006); Croatian (1979); Italian (1979); Dutch (1980); Icelandic (1991); Polish (1991, 2005); Swedish (2000); Spanish (2002)

Other Wiley Editorial Offices

John Wiley & Sons Inc., 111 River Street, Hoboken, NJ 07030, USA

Jossey-Bass, 989 Market Street, San Francisco, CA 94103-1741, USA

Wiley-VCH Verlag GmbH, Boschstr. 12, D-69469 Weinheim, Germany

John Wiley & Sons Australia Ltd, 33 Park Road, Milton, Queensland 4064, Australia

John Wiley & Sons (Asia) Pte Ltd, 2 Clementi Loop #02-01, Jin Xing Distripark, Singapore 129809

John Wiley & Sons Canada Ltd, 6045 Freemont Blvd, Mississauga, Ontario, L5R 4J3 Canada

Wiley also publishes its books in a variety of electronic formats. Some content that appears in print may not be available in electronic books.

Library of Congress Catalogoing-in-Publication Data

Gøtzsche, Peter C.
   Rational diagnosis and treatment : evidence-based clinical decision-making / Peter C. Gøtzsche. – 4th ed.
       p. ; cm.
   Rev. ed. of: Rational diagnosis and treatment / Henrik R. Wulff and Peter C. Gøtzsche. 3rd ed. 2000.
   Includes bibliographical references and index.
   ISBN 978-0-470-51503-7 (cloth : alk. paper)
  1. Clinical medicine–Decision making.   2. Evidence-based medicine.
3. Diagnosis–Philosophy.   4. Therapeutics–Philosophy.   I. Wulff, Henrik R. Rational diagnosis and treatment.   II. Title
   [DNLM: 1. Diagnosis.   2. Evidence-Based Medicine. WB 141 G687r 2007]
R723.5.W85 2007
616.07′5–dc22   2007032155

British Library Cataloguing in Publication Data

A catalogue record for this book is available from the British Library

ISBN 978 0 470 51503 7

Typeset in 10.5/12.5 pt Minion by Aptara, New Delhi, India
Printed and bound in Great Britain by TJ International, Padstow, Cornwall
This book is printed on acid-free paper responsibly manufactured from sustainable forestry in which at least two trees are planted for each one used for paper production.

Contents

Preface

'The aim of this book is to show that work at the bedside can present just as great an intellectual challenge and yield even more satisfaction than work in the laboratory. Clinical reasoning can be as rigorous and as logical as that in any other academic discipline. True, the information on which decisions are based contains many elements of uncertainty, but measurement of uncertainty can replace personal and intuitive experience so that reasons for a decision become explicit and subject to analysis'. This is a quotation from the foreword by Professor J. E. Lennard-Jones, MD, FRCP, to the first edition of this book, which was published in 1976.

The book was written to promote the principles of what is now called evidence-based medicine, which at that time was slowly gaining ground. Most clinicians knew little of the methodological details of, for instance, the randomized clinical trial and many were baffled even by those simple statistical expressions, such as P-values and confidence intervals, which increasingly found their way to the medical journals. Since that time much has changed. What was then new is now well accepted and regarded as something which ought to be taught at every medical school. A textbook, however, is still needed, and, therefore, I decided to publish a new edition of the book.

I am deeply indebted to Professor Emeritus Henrik R. Wulff, MD, who wrote the first two editions of this book and with whom I rewrote the third edition that came out in 2000. I have now revised the book again, taking into account the developments since its third edition, but the aim is the same. It presents an analysis of the foundation of the clinician's decisions when he or she faces the individual patient, and although it stresses the importance of stringent scientific thinking it does not ignore the human aspects of clinical work. It emphasizes the importance of clinical research, but the methodological intricacies are viewed from the perspective of the clinician who wishes to make rational diagnostic and therapeutic decisions, not from the point of view of the researcher.

The Danish edition of the book is part of the curriculum for medical students at the University of Copenhagen, and I hope that the updated English edition may be used for undergraduate teaching at other medical schools. I also hope that it will find its place in the continued education of medical practitioners.

Peter C. Gøtzsche, MD, MSc
Consultant Physician
Director of The Nordic Cochrane Centre
Rigshospitalet, Copenhagen

Peter C. Gøtzsche studied at the University of Copenhagen, Denmark, and at the universities in Uppsala and Lund, Sweden. He graduated as a scientist in biology and chemistry in 1974 and as a physician in 1984. He worked in the drug industry from 1975 till 1983, mainly with clinical trials and regulatory affairs, and as a clinician at hospitals in Copenhagen till 1995. In 1993, when Sir Iain Chalmers in Oxford, UK, founded The Cochrane Collaboration, Peter Gøtzsche established The Nordic Cochrane Centre. He has lectured in Theory of Medicine at the University of Copenhagen since 1988. His research is mainly clinically oriented and his thesis from 1990 is about bias in drug trials. He is a specialist in internal medicine.

Introduction

It is at the bedside we commence our labors and at the bedside we terminate them.

Knud Faber[1]

Medical students work their way through books on anatomy, physiology, microbiology, paediatrics, surgery and many other subjects; they have to read thousands of pages and to assimilate a multitude of facts mostly for one purpose, the practice of medicine.

Somewhere along the road the students must also be taught how to utilize all this theoretical knowledge for making the right diagnostic and therapeutic decisions, and this lesson is learnt on the wards and in the out-patient departments. We talk about clinical medicine, and the word clinical is derived from Greek *kline* = bed.

Theoretical knowledge is important and bedside teaching will always be indispensable, but nevertheless something is missing. I shall try to explain this by a number of examples.

The medical student may be shown a patient with a palpable liver and a serum aminotransferase level above normal, and the importance of these findings is discussed. That is useful, but sometimes the student is not taught to what extent physical findings are subject to inter- and intra-observer variation, how the normal range for a laboratory test is calculated, and what is understood by normality. Therefore, he may not be sufficiently critical when later he evaluates the clinical picture of one of his patients.[*]

---

[*] Anonymous persons are labeled 'he' in chapters with even numbers and 'she' in chapters with odd numbers.

The student may also see a patient with changed bowel habits who had a positive test for faecal occult blood, which led to further investigations and a diagnosis of colonic cancer. However, he may not know the difference between nosographic and diagnostic probabilities and the importance of the disease prevalence and the clinical spectrum, and, therefore, he will be unable to discuss the value of a diagnostic test. Later on, he may subject his patients to unnecessary diagnostic investigations and misinterpret the results.

Further, the student may see a patient with an acute attack of bronchial asthma and he may also observe that the attack quickly subsides when the patient is treated with a β-agonist. That may enhance the student's confidence in drug therapy, but his confidence may be exaggerated, if he has been taught nothing about the fallacies of uncontrolled experience. The asthma attack might have subsided anyway. Most of those drugs which are used today will be replaced by others within a few years, and the doctor who has not been schooled in critical thinking may well expose his patients to new, ineffective or even harmful treatments.

These examples show that the teaching of clinical medicine as a master–apprentice relationship has its limitations. The apprentice learns to imitate the decisions of the master but he does not learn to assess the basis for the decisions. In contemporary medicine many clinical decisions have such far-reaching consequences that, apart from bedside experience, medical students and doctors must be well acquainted with the theoretical foundation of clinical decision-making and the results of clinical research. The clinician who bases his decisions on the best available clinical evidence from systematic research and integrates this knowledge with his clinical expertise and the patients' preferences is practicing so-called 'evidence-based medicine'.[2]

Clinical decision theory, however, is not a well-defined discipline. Clinical reasoning is extremely complex and the thought processes leading to diagnostic decisions are not well understood. It is also difficult to get a good grasp of the knowledge which does exist since it must be pieced together from articles in journals of epidemiology, biostatistics, medical ethics and other specialized fields, as well as from a number of useful treatises.[2–19]

It is also important to realize that clinical medicine belongs both to the natural sciences and the humanities, and in this book I shall distinguish between the scientific and the humanistic aspects of clinical decisions. We shall deal mostly with the scientific aspect when we discuss the decision process, i.e. how the clinician makes his observations in the individual case, interprets the data and then endeavours to act as rationally as possible combining this information and his knowledge of the results of clinical research. But I am very much aware of the fact that the two aspects of clinical medicine are inseparable, and the book also comprises a chapter on the humanistic aspect, i.e. the understanding of the patient as a fellow human being and the analysis of the ethical aspects of the case.

The examples from the history of medicine that are interspersed in the text illustrate that clinical practice, to a much greater extent than is realized by most clinicians, is influenced by the ideas and traditions of previous generations of doctors. The lessons from history may help us to avoid repeating the mistakes of our predecessors. I have sought some primary sources, but most of the information comes second-hand through standard works on medical history.

In some of the chapters, clinical research methods are discussed in some detail, but the book has not been written for those who are actively engaged in, for instance, the assessment of new diagnostic and therapeutic methods. I only wish to guide the consumers of medical literature who have to be critical when they consider the practical consequences of the research of others. The busy clinician should remember that some knowledge of research methodology is a great time-saver as it enables the reader of medical journals to skip all those papers where the methods are obviously inadequate.

Critical reading requires some knowledge of biostatistics, but the reader need not have any prior knowledge of that topic. I only wish to introduce basic statistical reasoning and to show that the statistician's approach to clinical problems is closely linked to common sense and rational decision-making. A survey among Danish doctors revealed that their knowledge of fundamental statistical concepts (including P-values, standard errors and standard deviations) was so limited that they could not be expected to draw the right conclusions from those calculations that are reported in most medical papers. They realized themselves that this was an important problem.[20] There is no reason to believe that the situation is any better in other countries.

Although the book is not intended as a primer for researchers I hope to show on the following pages that there is a great need for clinical research both at hospitals and in general practice. Much of the research done today, also by clinicians, is laboratory-oriented and aims at exploring the causes and mechanisms of disease. Acquisition of that kind of knowledge is indispensable, also from a clinical point of view, as it may lead to the development of new diagnostic and therapeutic methods, but, before they are accepted, these new methods must be assessed critically in practice. Good clinical research can only be carried out by experienced clinicians, and research at the bedside presents as big an intellectual challenge as work in the laboratory and deserves the same respect.

I shall briefly present the structure of the book. In Chapter 1 the clinical decision process is compared to a flow chart. The first step is the collection of information, and the formal characteristics of the different kinds of data are discussed. This discussion continues in Chapter 2, which deals with the reliability and relevance of the clinical data. In Chapter 3 the disease classification, which is indispensable for recording clinical knowledge and experience, will be viewed from a historical, a theoretical and a practical perspective.

The diagnostic decision is discussed in Chapter 4. If the truth of the diagnosis can be established by independent means, it is possible to determine the efficacy of a diagnostic test. In other cases the true diagnosis remains concealed, and it then has little meaning from a logical standpoint to discuss whether a diagnosis is true or false.

The diagnosis is only a means to select the best treatment, and the next two chapters deal with the treatment decision. Chapter 5 explains what can be learned from previous generations of doctors, and the randomized clinical trial, which is the logical consequence of that lesson, is discussed in some detail in Chapter 6.

In Chapter 7 clinical medicine is viewed as a humanistic discipline, and the ethical aspects of clinical decisions is considered. Chapter 8 deals with research methods and biostatistics and is meant as a guide for readers of medical journals.

I hope that the detailed Index at the end of the book will prove helpful when those who use it for teaching purposes wish to find examples and information about specific topics.

Peter C. Gøtzsche

1

The Foundation of Clinical Decisions

Decision-making is ... something which concerns all of us, both as the makers of the choice and as sufferers of the consequences.

Lindley[21]

And what does 'outgrabe' mean? Well, 'outgribing' is something between bellowing and whistling, with a kind of sneeze in the middle: However, you'll hear it done, maybe – down in the wood yonder – and when you've once heard it you'll be quite content ...

Lewis Carrol in 'Through the Looking-Glass'

A person who feels ill will usually seek medical advice, and the doctor, having listened to her patient's complaints, will make those decisions which, to the best of her knowledge, will help the patient most. This sequence of events is not new. If a patient at the beginning of the thirteenth century had developed an acute fever, the physician would have prescribed some medicinal herb. White benedicta (blessed thistle) might have been the choice, because this herb was said to possess great healing powers when it was taken on an empty stomach and when Pater Noster and Ave Maria were recited three times.[22] If the incident had taken place 600 years later the doctor might have made a diagnosis of pneumonia using the newly invented stethoscope, and would probably have ordered blood letting, customary dietary measures and blistering (induced by dried, pulverized Spanish fly).

The situation today is just the same, except that the doctor has a choice between many more investigations and treatments, and that the decision may have much greater influence on the course of the disease, and, therefore, on the future life of the patient. The decision to treat a patient suffering from pneumonia with penicillin may ensure her survival when otherwise she might have died, and the decision not to do a lumbar puncture in a febrile patient may lead to her death from meningitis, although she could have been saved.

The clinical decision process

It is not so simple, however, that all positive decisions are beneficial and that all negative decisions – omissions – are harmful. All active treatments can produce harm (otherwise, they wouldn't be active) and many diagnostic procedures (e.g. liver biopsies and endoscopic examinations) are unpleasant and may cause complications. The clinician must carefully consider the consequences of her actions, both for the individual patient, and, as we shall discuss later, for the health service as a whole.

The clinical decision process is complex, but may be illustrated by a simple flow chart (Fig. 1.1). When contact between patient and doctor has been established, the data collection begins (Step 1). The doctor interrogates the patient, does a physical examination and asks for appropriate blood tests, X-ray examinations etc. When the examinations are concluded, the clinician assesses the data that have been collected and tries to make a diagnosis (Step 2). To do this she uses her *nosographic* knowledge, i.e. her knowledge of the manifestations of different diseases (nosography = disease description, derived from Greek *nosos* = disease).

A diagnosis may be more or less certain, and the clinician has to ask herself whether or not the diagnosis is sufficiently well founded to proceed to treatment (Step 3). If the answer is 'no', the process returns to Step 1 and the investigations continue. If the answer is 'yes' the clinician proceeds to Step 4.

At this point she must once again draw on her nosographic knowledge, this time of the prognosis of the disease and the effect of different treatments. She chooses the treatment that is considered likely to help the patient most, and if the patient progresses as expected, the process comes to an end (Step 5).

This presentation is, of course, greatly simplified and frequently the decisions proceed in a different way. Sometimes the patient does not respond to treatment as expected, and the diagnosis must be revised; and sometimes it is necessary to institute treatment before the final diagnosis is made, as, for instance, in cases of haemorrhagic shock when treatment is started before the site of the bleeding is known. The flow chart also ignores the fact that in chronic diseases clinicians

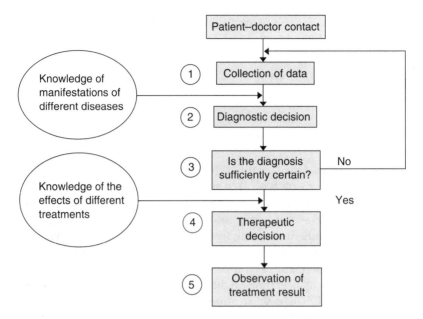

Fig. 1.1 Flow chart illustrating the clinical decision process.

must consider the long-term effects of their treatments, and the presentation does not take into account that doctors concern themselves not only with treatment, but also with prophylaxis.

Therefore, the flow chart in Fig. 1.1 is by no means universally valid, but it may serve as a framework for a systematic analysis of the decision process.

Clinical reasoning may be *deductive* or *empirical*. Clinicians reason deductively when they base their treatment decisions on deductions from theoretical knowledge of disease mechanisms and the mechanism of action of different drugs, whereas they reason empirically when their decision is based on experience that has been gained from the treatment of other patients. When a clinician recommends a β_2-agonist for the treatment of asthma, her reasoning is deductive if she argues that the symptoms are caused by bronchoconstriction and that β_2-agonists decrease this. Her reasoning is empirical, however, if she recommends steroid inhalations because randomized trials have shown a good and sustained effect with little harm.

Deductive and *empirical* reasoning constitute the scientific component of clinical decision-making (if we use the word scientific in its narrow sense, i.e. 'pertaining to the natural sciences'), but added to this is the humanistic component which comprises reasoning based on an *understanding* of the patient as a fellow human being, and *ethical* reasoning based on ethical norms (see Chapter 7). Thus, clinical decision-making is a synthesis of four types of reasoning.

Clinical data

A house physician at a medical unit reports to a registrar that she has just seen a new patient who presents with a red and swollen left lower leg and tenderness of the calf. The registrar accepts the suggestion that anticoagulant treatment is instituted in order to prevent progression of the surmised deep venous thrombosis. However, another houseman who has also seen the patient objects. It is true that the leg is red and swollen, but the demarcation of the erythema is sharp, the affected skin is raised compared with the adjoining normal skin, and the patient has a small ulceration on the foot. The registrar now correctly diagnoses erysipelas and changes the treatment to penicillin. The example illustrates the well-known danger involved when decisions are made by a doctor who has not examined the patient herself. Both diagnosis and treatment depend on the collected data and no amount of professional knowledge can compensate for incorrect information. Therefore, it is not possible to attempt an analysis of diagnostic and therapeutic decision-making until the information that is used for the decisions has been analysed in detail, but unfortunately this analysis is hampered by the fact that many of the terms that we generally use are vague and ill defined.

In this book I shall use the term *clinical data* to denote all those data about the individual patient which are relevant for the decision process, and collectively these data are said to constitute the patient's *clinical picture*. Consequently, the clinical data in this wide sense comprise both the data recorded at the bedside (symptoms and signs), i.e. the truly clinical data, and the results of laboratory investigations, i.e. the so-called paraclinical data. Further, the clinical data (and the clinical picture) include negative findings, such as 'the lack of neck stiffness' in a febrile patient.

I shall use the following definitions of the different types of clinical data:

- *Subjective symptoms.* These are the sensations noted by the patient (e.g. pain, clouded vision and dizziness) and the patient's mood (e.g. depression and anxiety).

- *Objective symptoms.* This term signifies all observations made by the patient or the relatives concerning the patient's body and its products, e.g. swollen ankles, blood in the urine or an epileptic attack.

- *Physical signs.* These comprise all those observations that are made by the doctor during the physical examination, e.g. a cardiac murmur, swollen lymph nodes or jaundice. Some of the recorded 'signs', such as tenderness, dysaesthesia or loss of central vision of one eye, fall into a special group. They are subjective symptoms that are only noticed by the patient during the physical examination, and they may appropriately be called *provoked symptoms.*

- *Paraclinical data.* They include all laboratory results, and the results of all examinations not done by the clinician herself, such as blood analyses or radiological and histological findings. Paraclinical data may be either *descriptive,* e.g. the shadow on a chest X-ray, or *quantitative,* e.g. the blood glucose concentration.

The patient's record will also contain other data that may be of paramount importance, e.g. information about occupation, family life, previous illnesses, medication, smoking, drinking and other habits.

The erysipelas case illustrated that incomplete or unreliable information may easily lead the decision process astray, and it is worthwhile considering how the clinical data come to the clinician's attention. We may for this purpose distinguish between three types of data:

1. The symptoms that make the patients seek medical advice;

2. The data that are revealed by the routine questioning and the routine investigation of the patient;

3. The data that are the results of diagnostic tests that are carried out to confirm or exclude various diagnostic possibilities.

The first type of data may be labelled the *iatrotropic symptoms* (from Greek *iatros* = doctor and *trope* = turn).[3] They are the subjective and objective symptoms that make the patient turn to her doctor as opposed to the non-iatrotropic symptoms which are only disclosed during the taking of the history. In the same way one may distinguish between iatrotropic and non-iatrotropic cases of a disease. A patient who sends for a doctor because of a high temperature and who, during history taking admits having epigastric pain, may represent an iatrotropic case of pneumonia and a non-iatrotropic case of duodenal ulcer.

Non-iatrotropic cases may also be diagnosed during a routine medical 'check-up' or at mass screening for some disease, e.g. tuberculosis.

Iatrotropic symptoms are of particular importance as they usually represent that problem which the doctor, in the eyes of the patient, has to solve, and they ought to be given particular prominence, especially in hospital notes. Nowadays it is not rare in hospital practice that the investigations bring some unexpected findings to light which then lead to further investigations along a side-track. After a while the whole staff is interested in, say, the immunoglobulin pattern, and nobody remembers why the patient was admitted. Only on the day on which the patient is discharged will she say, 'But you have not done anything about my backache!'. The advanced specialization of hospital departments invites the occurrence of such incidents. If a patient presents a complex clinical picture, the subspecialized physician may more or less consciously emphasize those clinical data which pertain to her own field of interest, whereas the remaining data are treated more lightly.

A symptom may become iatrotropic for a number of reasons. One patient with abdominal pain may ask to see her doctor because she is afraid of cancer while somebody else with the same complaint may be worried about losing her job, and in other cases the reason for the visit is not directly related to the symptoms. The patient may have felt a lump in the breast which she dares not mention, but hopes that the doctor will find, or she may have problems at work or at home which made her contact her doctor on the pretext of some mild symptom, which under normal circumstances she would have accepted. Personal problems of any kind may lower the *threshold of iatrotropy*.

The second type of data are recorded routinely from all patients. In hospital practice they comprise answers to standard questions during history taking, the results of the ordinary physical examination and some simple paraclinical tests, such as haemoglobin determination and urine analysis. The routine history taking and examination are to a large extent determined by tradition and from time to time they must be brought up to date. It is no longer necessary in some countries to ask all elderly patients whether they have had rheumatic fever or diphtheria, but it is important to ask detailed questions about their social network and their living conditions. Perhaps the dangers of working with organic solvents would have been detected earlier if the notes contained more routine information about occupation and working conditions.

The third type of data are those collected during the diagnostic process, which begins as soon as the iatrotropic symptoms have been recorded. The clinician will, for instance, ask a jaundiced patient if she has had abdominal pain and or if she has travelled abroad, and such specific questions may well be likened to diagnostic tests, which aim at confirming or excluding different diagnostic possibilities. In other words, the process passes through the loop in the flow chart (Fig. 1.1) many times already during the taking of the history.

Scales of measurement

Clinical data have many characteristics that are not peculiar to medicine, and I shall now consider the classification of data in general terms, using nonmedical examples. There are three levels of measurement scales:[23] the nominal scale, the ordinal scale and the interval scale.

At a music lesson, a recording of a short passage from an orchestral work is played and the children are asked to identify the solo instrument at a particular moment. Each child is asked to indicate her reply on a list of all the instruments of the orchestra. Such a list, which is used to classify qualitative observations in a series of named categories, is called a *nominal scale*, which, from a formal point of view, must fulfil three conditions. Firstly, each category or class must be well defined, and we shall see later that this requirement in particular causes great difficulties in clinical medicine. Secondly, the classification must be exclusive, meaning that no observation must belong to more than one category, and thirdly the classification must be exhaustive, which means that all observations to be classified must belong to one of the categories. It is often possible to reduce a nominal scale to fewer classes. In the present example one might have used four classes (strings, woodwind, brass and percussion) or even two classes ('stringed instruments' and 'other instruments'). A scale consisting of only two classes is called a *binary scale*.

Observations may be more refined. In 1806 the British admiral Sir Francis Beaufort constructed a scale for the measurement of wind force. The scale, which consists of 13 classes, is shown in Table 1.1. This is an example of an *ordinal scale*, and although it must have formed the basis for important decisions in the course of history, it has its limitations. We may take it for granted that a Force 10 is greater than, say, a Force 8, and that a Force 3 is greater than a Force 1, but we must not presuppose that the difference between Force 10 and Force 8 is the same as the difference between Force 3 and Force 1. That was revealed (as shown in Table 1.1) when it became possible to measure the wind force in m/s. To measure on an ordinal scale is like using an unevenly stretched elastic tape measure, and therefore it makes little sense calculating the 'mean windforce'. An ordinal scale may also be reduced to a binary scale, which would be the case if we only distinguished between 'windy weather' and 'calm weather'.

Table 1.1 Beaufort scale of wind force. Specifications for use on land. The numbers in brackets indicate the wind force in m/s.

---

0. *Calm.* Smoke rises vertically (0–0.2).
1. *Light air.* Direction of wind shown by smoke drift, but not by wind wanes (0.3–1.5).
2. *Light breeze.* Wind felt on face; leaves rustle; ordinary wane moved by wind (1.6–3.3).
3. *Gentle breeze.* Leaves and small twists in constant motion; wind extends light flag (3.4–5.4).
4. *Moderate breeze.* Raises dust and loose paper; small branches are moved (5.5–7.9).
5. *Fresh breeze.* Small trees in leaf begin to sway; crested wavelets form on inland waters (8.0–10.7).
6. *Strong breeze.* Large branches in motion; whistling heard in telegraph wires; umbrellas used with difficulty (10.8–13.8).
7. *Moderate gale.* Whole trees in motion; inconvenience felt in walking against wind (13.9–17.1).
8. *Fresh gale.* Breaks twigs off trees; generally impedes progress (17.2–20.7).
9. *Strong gale.* Slight structural damage occurs (chimney pots and slates removed) (20.8–24.4).
10. *Whole gale.* Seldom experienced inland; trees uprooted; considerable structural damage occurs (24.5–28.4).
11. *Storm.* Very rarely experienced; accompanied by widespread damage (28.5–32.6).
12. *Hurricane.* Disastrous results (>32.6).

The *ranking* of data also provides measurements on an ordinal scale. School children may, for instance, be ranked from the top to the bottom of the form according to their proficiency, but once again one cannot assume that the difference between the proficiency of, say, numbers 5 and 6, is the same as that between numbers 6 and 7.

The *interval scale* represents the highest level of measurement. Weighing an object on a balance or the wind force in m/s may serve as examples. In these cases the scale is continuous and the interval, which is constant along the scale, is chosen to suit the precision of the measuring instrument. It may be 1 g for an ordinary letter balance and much less for an analytical balance. Interval scales may also be discontinuous (discrete). The number of patients in a ward may be 27 or 28, but not 27.5.

Usually, an interval scale is also a *ratio scale*. For instance, an object weighing 28 g is twice as heavy as an object weighing 14 g. Only measurements on a scale with an arbitrary zero point form an exception. Water having a temperature of 28 °C is not twice as warm as water having a temperature of 14 °C.

Measurements on an interval scale may be reduced to an ordinal or a binary scale. We may, for instance, measure objects in grams, but for some purposes we may confine ourselves to distinguishing between very heavy, heavy and light objects or just between heavy and light objects. This terminology is useful for the analysis of clinical data.

Taking the history

Often the patient is not able to give a concise account of her complaints and the following example of a conversation between a patient and her doctor may serve as an example.

Doctor:	'Good morning, Mrs N.N. What is the trouble?'
Patient:	'I have had an uncomfortable feeling in my chest recently.'
D:	'Have you got a pain?'
P:	'I feel as though I cannot breathe.'
D:	'When does this happen? When you exert yourself or when you are resting?'
P:	'It only happens when I am working; when I do the cleaning I have to keep stopping to get my breath.'
D:	'I remember you live on the second floor; how do you get on going up the stairs?'
P:	'I take it slowly, but I have to wait on each landing'.
D:	'How long has it been troubling you?'
P:	'Ever since Christmas, but it got worse.'

This piece of conversation shows how the questioning progresses. The patient presents a vague complaint, 'an uncomfortable feeling in the chest', and it takes the doctor a couple of questions to be sure that the problem is dyspnoea on exertion. One may imagine that the doctor has in her mind a nominal scale of all possible symptoms, and that she is trying to refer her patient's complaint to one of these named categories. Classification on a nominal scale, however, requires that all categories are well defined, and unfortunately most symptoms do not fulfil this requirement. All doctors may agree that the symptom angina pectoris suggests arteriosclerotic heart disease, but if participants in postgraduate medical courses are asked how they define the symptom, then the replies vary. Some say that it is necessary that the pain only occurs during exertion and others demand that the pain has a typical radiation. It always provokes heated discussion when doctors are asked to define common medical terms; there is immediate disagreement with an admixture of aggression, as everybody believes that her interpretation is the right one.

The patient in the example had dyspnoea, and that term is also ambiguous as it is used to describe both a subjective symptom (shortness of breath) and a physical sign (visibly laboured respiration). I shall return to the problem of definitions several times in this book, and I shall also point out that it does not matter so much which defining criteria are chosen, as long as there is mutual agreement. Authors of textbooks could do much to bring about such standardization.

It is best always to use neutral medical terms, i.e. terms that do not imply the cause of the complaint, and to avoid expressions such as ulcer dyspepsia, pleural pain and biliary colics. Such *diagnostic data transformation* is often found in medical notes and it may prejudice the clinician against other diagnostic possibilities. One should not attempt to make a diagnosis until the necessary data have been collected.

When the complaint has been named and classified its degree of severity must be assessed. In the example, the doctor extracted the information that the patient had to stop from time to time while doing her housework and that she must rest on each landing going upstairs. The severity of the symptoms can often be measured on an ordinal scale using expressions like mild, moderate and severe, but first it is necessary to define, as exactly as possible, the individual classes. We may, for instance, talk about mild dyspnoea if it does not limit normal activity, moderate dyspnoea if it limits but does not prevent normal activity, and severe dyspnoea if it prevents normal activity. Such an ordinal scale with predefined classes is often called a *rating scale*, and in the example the patient's dyspnoea is rated as moderate. The severity of other symptoms as, for instance, abdominal pain in gastric ulcer patients may be assessed in exactly the same way: The patient notices the pain but continues working normally, her working capacity is reduced, or she stops working.

In these examples the severity was graded according to an ordinal scale with defined classes, but the severity of the symptoms in a particular patient may also be assessed over time by simple ranking. A patient may say: 'I am feeling better than at the last visit, but I am not as well as I was this summer'.

A more refined method has been suggested for the measurement of pain intensity in, for instance, rheumatoid arthritis. The patients are asked to mark the degree of their complaint on a so-called *visual analogue scale*, i.e. a line, usually 100 mm long, ranging from 'no pain' to 'pain as bad as pain can be' (Fig. 1.2).[24] Usually, however, this method cannot be recommended. Everybody knows what it means to suffer no pain, but the other end of the scale is left to the patient's imagination, and in practice patients may be reluctant to commit themselves when they are shown the line.

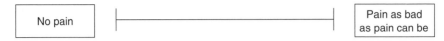

Fig. 1.2 Visual analogue scale for measuring pain.

The method also invites statistical problems. It is tempting to believe that the visual analogue scale is an interval scale and that it permits measurement of pain in mm, but that is not the case. It is only an ordinal scale, as it cannot be taken for granted that a difference of 10 mm at the lower end of the scale corresponds to the same difference in pain intensity as a difference of 10 mm at the higher end of the scale. Therefore, it makes little sense to calculate, for instance, mean and standard deviation, which presuppose an interval scale, and instead one should use ordinal scale statistics (with calculation of median and quantiles) as explained in Chapter 8. It has been shown that the grading of pain in rheumatoid arthritis, using a simple rating scale with four or five classes, is more sensitive than measurements on a visual analogue scale.[25]

Finally, the symptom must be assessed chronologically. In the example the patient had suffered dyspnoea 'since Christmas' and this information is recorded as the number of months or weeks, i.e. on an interval scale. In the case of intermittent symptoms the chronological assessment also includes the duration of attacks and the intervals between them.

The physical examination

The physical examination, as it is performed today, originated in France at the beginning of the nineteenth century at which time the so-called Paris School of pathological anatomy was flourishing. Anatomical and clinical observations were correlated, and it became the task of the clinician, by means of the physical examination, to make those diagnoses that were known from autopsy studies.

Examination of the lungs and heart was developed at that time. Corvisart (1755–1821), Napoleon's physician, made percussion a routine examination and Laënnec (1781–1826) developed auscultation by means of the stethoscope. It is said that once Laënnec had to examine an obese female patient, he could not feel the apex beat and in order not to apply his ear to her chest in an unseemly manner he rolled a sheaf of paper into a cylinder. Auscultation had its golden age before the introduction of radiology, electrocardiography and echography, but it is still of considerable importance. In general practice the decision whether or not to treat a febrile patient with penicillin may depend on the result of the examination of the chest.

Unfortunately, the terminology that we use to describe our findings is chaotic. Anybody who spends a little time looking up the clinical signs in pneumonia, asthma and bronchitis in different textbooks will be surprised by the plethora of undefined terms. Perhaps we should confine ourselves to talking about coarse bubbling sounds (typically in chronic bronchitis), wheezing (in asthma), fine bubbling sounds (in pneumonia and congestive heart disease), and friction rubs (in pleurisy).

It is possible that computer technology will improve the situation by the introduction of educational programmes where the student sees the examination of the patient on the screen and at the same time hears what the physician hears in her stethoscope. In that way ostensive definitions, i.e. definition by demonstration of typical cases, may replace the usual verbal definitions.

In hospital practice, chest auscultation is part of the routine physical examination, but other clinical examinations are only done on those patients who present certain clinical pictures, e.g. palpation of the temporal artery in patients with pyrexia of unknown origin or examination for ruptured ligaments after a knee trauma. Such examinations represent diagnostic tests that are carried out on the suspicion of a particular diagnosis.

Paraclinical findings

Typically, paraclinical findings are the results of all those tests and observations that are made in the 'paraclinical' departments, i.e. departments of pathology, clinical chemistry, radiology etc. (but they may also be said to include those simple laboratory tests which are done by the clinicians themselves). They serve a clinical purpose and, therefore, they are included when in this book I use the term clinical data or talk about the patient's clinical picture.

Radiological, scintigraphic and histological findings are examples of descriptive, paraclinical data. They must, just like symptoms and physical signs, be classified by means of a nominal scale with well-defined classes (e.g. different types of colonic polyps), and they may be graded on an ordinal scale (e.g. slight, moderate or severe dysplasia).

Paraclinical observations are usually considered more objective, and therefore more reliable than those observations that are made at the bedside. This may often be true, but clinicians should be aware of the fact that, for instance, X-ray reports may be biased by the information on the request form, in which case the paraclinical observation may just help to sustain a wrong diagnosis. In order to solve this problem, the suggestion has been made that the paraclinical diagnostician should receive no information about the patient's clinical picture, but that is of course quite unrealistic. A radiologist, for instance, must know which clinical problem she is expected to solve, just as the physician doing a clinical examination will take into account whether the patient is febrile, has abdominal pain or presents other symptoms. However, unnecessary diagnostic data transformation is to be avoided. The radiologist who sees a consolidation in one lung should strive at a neutral description of this finding, and she should not write 'pneumonia' if it is noted on the request form that the patient has a high temperature, but something else if the temperature is normal. The radiologist's expert advice is, of course, needed when the clinician considers various diagnostic possibilities, but ideally the synthesis of the radiological findings and the rest of the information about the patient should take place after the initial description of the films, for instance, at a joint X-ray conference. In clinical research, however, it is essential that the X-ray films are read by a radiologist who has no knowledge of the other components of the clinical picture.

Histological reports present a special problem as the pathoanatomical diagnosis frequently also represents the patient's diagnosis, simply because the disease classification to a large extent is anatomically orientated. It is, however, necessary to be aware of the fact that doctors representing different specialties sometimes attach very different meanings to the same terms. Gastritis is a good example. Particularly in the past, general practitioners have often used this term as a diagnostic label for patients with upper abdominal dyspepsia. Gastroenterologists use the term to denote certain endoscopic findings, and pathologists only talk about gastritis if histological sections of a biopsy show inflammatory or atrophic changes.

A different example is provided by the words 'acute' and 'chronic'. To the clinician 'acute' means 'of sudden onset' and 'chronic' is used in the sense 'persistent', whereas to the pathologist 'acute' is synonymous with 'infiltrated with polymorphs' and 'chronic' denotes 'infiltrated with round cells'. A rectal biopsy from a patient with ulcerative colitis usually presents 'acute inflammatory changes' in spite of the fact that the patient may have had the disease for many years.

The concentrations of different substances in the patient's blood are typical examples of quantitative paraclinical data, representing measurements on an interval scale. Such results are usually less ambiguous than the descriptive data, but the clinician should remember that methods of analysis vary and that results from different laboratories may not be comparable.

Global assessments

Up to now I have considered the assessment of the individual components of the clinical picture, but often clinical decisions are based not only on the presence or absence of a particular symptom or sign, but also on a global assessment of the patient's condition. The general practitioner who visits a child with a high temperature may not be able to make a specific diagnosis and then she will rely on her global evaluation of the child's condition. A child who 'looks ill' may be admitted to hospital at once, whereas the child who seems relatively unaffected will be observed at home.

Global assessments are also essential when clinicians assess the effect of their treatments, both in the daily routine and in clinical research. Therefore, it is unfortunate when papers in medical journals concerning the effect of cancer chemotherapy only report the effect on survival. It is, of course, important to know the average number of days that the patients survived when they received different treatments, but this information ought to be supplemented with global assessments of their condition during the course of the disease. It must be reported how they felt, what they were able to do, and how the harms of the treatments affected them.

It may be useful for research purposes, but also in daily clinical practice, to formalize such global assessments by calculating a *clinical index*[11] and for that purpose one may use simple rating scales or more complex scoring systems. The rating scales are constructed much like the Beaufort scale (see Table 1.1). The number of classes may vary, but, if a simple five-point scale is used, the patients may record at the end of the treatment period (provided it is so short that they can remember how their condition was before treatment) whether they feel much better, a little better, the same, a little worse or much worse. The ratings may also be observer ratings, i.e. ratings done by the clinician, but in both cases it is important, as Beaufort did, to define the classes as well as possible.

The New York Heart Association (NYHA) classification of the functional capacity of patients with cardiac incompetence is a good example of a rating scale. It uses the following criteria (abbreviated):

1. No limitation of physical activity;

2. Ordinary physical activity results in fatigue, palpitation or dyspnoea;

3. Less than ordinary activity causes fatigue, palpitation or dyspnoea;

4. Symptoms at rest.[26]

In other cases the components of the global assessment cannot be measured on the same scale, and then one must rate each component independently and afterwards calculate a total score. A well-known example is the Apgar score for assessing the state of the newborn. Here the heart rate, respiratory effort, muscle tone, response to stimuli and colour are rated independently as 0, 1 or 2, and the total score is calculated by simple addition of the five ratings.[27] Other scoring systems, however, are much more complicated. Some anaesthesiologists, for instance, use the APACHE score to assess the prognosis of critically ill patients, which includes both a clinical assessment and a large number of laboratory tests (e.g. electrolytes, arterial pH and the white blood cell count).[28]

The calculation of clinical indices may be useful, but it is a condition that they make sense from a clinical point of view, and that is not always the case. More than 70 different methods for assessing the treatment effect in rheumatoid arthritis have been used, and some of them make little sense.[29] Previously, Ritchie's index was often calculated. Here the doctor palpates a number of joints, records the pain response on a rating scale from 0 to 3, adds up the results and calculates the total score. In other studies the doctor simply counts the number of tender or swollen joints. When these methods are used, two patients, one with a severe pain in one or two joints and another with a slight pain in a larger number of joints, may receive the same score, although, obviously, the former patient is much more incapacitated than the latter. In trials of schizophrenia, more than 600 different scales have been used[30] and, obviously, they cannot all have been meaningful.

Global assessments made by the patients themselves by means of a visual analogue scale are also of little use. The end points of the scale are defined as 'the best imaginable' and the 'worst imaginable' condition which means that their definition is left to the imagination of the patient. In most cases it is better to use simple rating scales with few classes.[25]

No matter which method is used, it must be remembered that we are dealing with measurements on an ordinal scale, and, although it is often done, it makes little sense to calculate the mean and the standard deviation (Chapter 8). Complex clinical indices are sometimes referred to as *quality of life* measurements, but this term should not be used in this context (Chapter 7).

2
Reliability and Relevance of Clinical Data

On the basis of this exercise there were clearly considerable difficulties in achieving agreement between experts. In fact it appeared that if one had involved a fifth interpreter there might well have been no finding on which all observers would have agreed.

Higgins, Cochrane and Thomas[31]

Why did I ask for this pathological investigation? Now that I have the result in my hand, I have no idea why I ordered it. It has, as far as I can see, no possible bearing on the case. Whatever the result, it would not influence the diagnosis or the treatment.

Lancet[32]

The quotations illustrate that we must always consider the reliability of the clinical data that we record, as well as the reason for recording them. This is the topic of the present chapter, but first it is necessary to introduce a suitable terminology.

Observations are *reliable* if they are both *reproducible* and *accurate*. Imagine a serum sample in which the concentration of the substance 'imaginate' is exactly 80 mmol/L. We send portions of this sample to four different laboratories and ask them to determine the imaginate concentration. Each laboratory performs 10 analyses of their sample, and the results are shown in Table 2.1.

In laboratory A practically all the results are correct which means that the reliability of the analysis is good. In contrast, the results from laboratories

Table 2.1   Results obtained when a serum sample with a true imaginate content of 80 mmol/L was analysed at four different laboratories A, B, C and D. The mean values are 80, 80, 90 and 88 mmol/L.

Laboratory			
A	B	C	D
80	81	91	78
79	75	90	91
81	85	89	87
80	73	89	95
80	87	91	88
81	80	90	84
80	82	89	79
80	69	90	92
80	78	91	94
79	89	90	89

B and C are unreliable, but in two different ways. Those from laboratory B are unreliable as regards their *reproducibility* (also called *precision*), since the measurements vary unpredictably around the true value. They are subject to random variation, but, if we calculate the mean, we get approximately the true value. The results from laboratory C are unreliable with respect to their *accuracy* since they are all too high. They are subject to a *systematic error* (*bias*), but they are reproducible. The results from laboratory D are unreliable in both respects.

These terms are useful for discussing the reliability of clinical data measured on an interval scale, but they are also applicable to observations on a binary scale. Imagine, for instance, that several radiologists look at the same X-ray films. If some of them say that the films are normal while others disagree, we must conclude that the reliability is poor. The reproducibility would only have been maximal if they had all agreed, but even that would not have proved that they were right. Perhaps all of them made the same mistake.

We shall now consider in greater detail the reliability of clinical data measured on an interval scale, an ordinal scale and a binary (nominal) scale, but for good reasons I shall not discuss the reliability of subjective symptoms. Patients' statements about their sensations are of course, very important, but obviously it makes little sense to discuss their reproducibility, as it is futile to ask the same questions again and again, and it is also impossible to prove their accuracy, except indirectly, if some objective observation explains the complaints. The observation of a gastric ulcer at endoscopy may, for instance, be said to confirm the sensation of abdominal pain. Nevertheless, one should aim at maximum reliability by defining different symptoms as well as possible and by using a thorough, neutral questioning technique.

Clinical data on an interval scale

Suppose that the biochemist in laboratory B had performed not just 10, but several hundred analyses of the imaginate concentration in the serum sample. These results might be shown in a bar chart (histogram), where each bar represents the number of analyses that give a particular result (Fig. 2.1a). It is seen that the histogram has assumed the shape of a bell, which, apart from the serration, resembles the curve in Fig. 2.1b.

The curve is defined by a mathematical equation, which is also shown in Fig. 2.1b, and it is not quite unexpected that the histogram resembles this particular mathematically defined curve. Suppose that the imaginate analysis is very complicated and sensitive. When, for instance, the temperature is a little too high the result of the analysis will also be a little too high, when it is too low the result will be too low; when pH is a little too high the result will be too low, etc. If in this way the analysis is subject to a large number of small errors which either pull the result up or down, then it is to be expected for mathematical reasons that the distribution of the results will be symmetrically bell-shaped, approaching the theoretical curve in Fig. 2.1b. Usually, the small errors neutralize one another, which has the effect that we obtain many results near the mean and only few results in the 'tails' of the curve. This mathematically defined distribution was described by Carl Friedrich Gauss (1777–1855) when he was 17 years old and may therefore be called the *Gaussian distribution*. It is also called the *normal distribution*.

If the biochemist wanted to publish his results, he might include the bar chart in his paper, but he may also feel that it is sufficient to communicate the mean and the standard deviation. The *standard deviation(s)* is calculated by the following formula:

$$s = \sqrt{\frac{\sum (x - \overline{x})^2}{n - 1}}$$

where n is the number of observations, x the individual observations and $\overline{x}$ the mean.

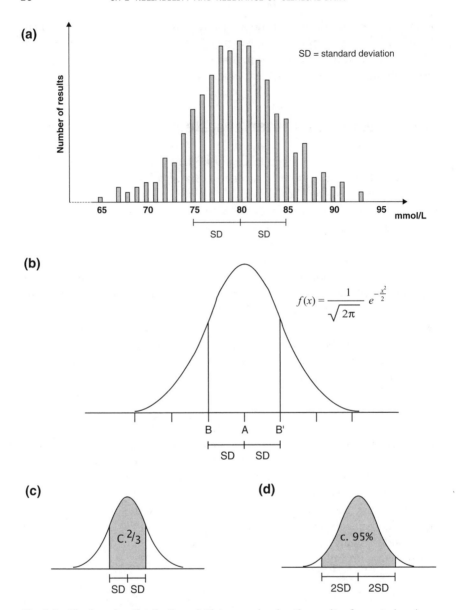

Fig. 2.1   The Gaussian distribution. a) Histogram showing the results of repeated analyses of the imaginate content in the same sample. b) The mathematically defined Gaussian distribution curve (and the formula for the curve if mean = 0 and the standard deviation = 1). c) Mean ± one standard deviation cuts off approximately two-thirds of the area below the Gaussian curve. d) Mean ± two standard deviations cuts off approximately 95% of the area below the Gaussian curve.

Once again it is not necessary to worry about the mathematics, but let us just assume that the standard deviation, when it is calculated according to this formula, is found to be 5 mmol/L. It is much more important to understand what this result really means, and for that purpose the interval mean ± one standard deviation has been marked in Fig. 2.1a and Fig. 2.1b. In Fig. 2.1a it reaches from 75 to 85 mmol/L and in Fig. 2.1b from B to B′. We may then draw perpendiculars through these points and it will be seen that they intersect the curve at its points of inflexion, i.e. the points where the curve changes from being convex to being concave. Thus, the mean tells us where the top of the curve is, and the standard deviation tells us where the points of inflection are located.

These considerations are of great practical interest, as it is possible (by means of the equation) to calculate that the area under the curve between the perpendiculars, i.e. the area corresponding to mean ± one standard deviation, constitutes approximately two-thirds of the total area (Fig. 2.1c). Consequently, it must be expected in this case that two thirds of the results fell within the region 80 ± 5 mmol/L or between 75 and 85 mmol/L. Similarly, it can be calculated that the area corresponding to mean ± two standard deviations makes up approximately 95% of the total area. Therefore, approximately 95% of the results of the analyses ranged from 70 to 90 mmol/L (Fig. 2.1d).

Assuming that the distribution of the results is approximately Gaussian, the standard deviation may be used to indicate the reproducibility of quantitative analyses. Or, alternatively, one may calculate the *variation coefficient*, which is just the standard deviation as a percentage of the mean. This calculation has the advantage that the result is independent of the unit of measurement. In most cases of repeated measurements of the same sample the Gaussian assumption is reasonable, but it is quite possible to imagine an analysis where the errors produce a skew distribution, and then it makes little sense to report the standard deviation.

In this example the analysis was accurate, as the mean of all the repeated analyses equalled the true concentration. If that had not been the case, i.e. if the analysis had been subject to a systematic error as in laboratories C and D (Table 2.1), the difference between the calculated mean concentration and the true concentration could be used to indicate the degree of bias.

Blood pressure measurements are done at the bedside and may therefore be regarded as physical signs, but, since they are recorded on an interval scale, they may also be discussed in this context. If several doctors measure the blood pressure of the same patient, using an ordinary sphygmomanometer, the reproducibility will not be perfect, as they will position the cuff a little differently and as they will not register the change in the sound of the pulse beat at exactly the same time. The results may resemble those in Fig. 2.1a, but probably they will also reveal a particular type of bias. It is well known that there is a tendency to record the blood pressure as multiples of five, for which reason it is more likely that a manometer reading will be, say, 150 or 155 than 152. The accuracy of the readings could be determined by intra-arterial blood pressure measurement.

Measurement of the body temperature illustrates well that the reliability should be measured in a clinical practice setting and not in a laboratory. In Denmark, we gave up using rectal mercury thermometers many years ago, and instead we introduced electronic oral thermometers. They gave reproducible and accurate results when they were dipped into warm water, but in practice they proved very unreliable compared to rectal readings.[33] Then, electronic temperature measurement in the ear was introduced, but it was shown many years later that infrared ear thermometry would fail to diagnose fever in one-third of children with a rectal temperature of 38 °C or above.[34] The reliability of these methods ought to have been tested in a clinical setting before they were introduced, but that was not done.

The reliability of the imaginate analysis would also depend on the circumstances. It would undoubtedly have been much lower if the laboratory had done the repeated analyses of the sample as part of the daily routine on successive days. Then they would have been carried out by different laboratory technicians, and it might have been necessary to use a succession of batches of the reagents.

Clinical data on an ordinal scale

Measurements on an ordinal scale play a very important role, both in clinical practice and in clinical research. As explained in the preceding chapter, simple rating scales may be used to grade the severity of symptoms and clinical indices to make global assessments, but such methods should not be introduced unless it has been shown that the reproducibility is satisfactory. Unfortunately, the reproducibility is often poor. Usually, the accuracy cannot be assessed, except indirectly, if the global assessment serves a diagnostic or prognostic purpose. Then one may correlate the clinical index to the diagnosis or prognosis of the individual patients.

Clinical data on a binary scale

Descriptive paraclinical findings

In the 1950s, a very large study was carried out, where 10 doctors read almost 15 000 small chest films taken as part of a screening programme for tuberculosis among college students.[35] The doctors were asked whether the films were positive or negative, a positive film being one which raised the suspicion of pulmonary tuberculosis to such an extent that the reader would like to see a larger chest film of the patient. In all, 1307 films were interpreted as positive by one or more observers, and by an elaborate decision process involving a panel of expert radiologists it was decided in the end that for 249 patients the films were truly positive in the sense that these patients required further examination. A further analysis of the results showed that, on average, each reader interpreted 39% of the truly positive films as negative and 1.2% of the truly negative films as positive. The use of the expressions 'truly positive' and 'truly negative' give the impression that the study's authors had assessed the accuracy of the readings, but of course that was not the case, as nobody can decide the truth of the statement that a patient is in need of further examination to exclude or confirm pulmonary tuberculosis. In fact, only 8 of the 249 students were found to have active tuberculosis, and the study only provides the information that the reproducibility was rather poor, or, using another expression, that the *inter-observer agreement* was low.

These researchers also carried out an *intra-observer study* in which the same observers read the same films twice[36] and this time the reproducibility was somewhat better.

These projects raised a lot of discussion at the time. They inspired further studies, which gave similar results, and there can be no doubt that the reproducibility of descriptive clinical data is an important issue. The quotation which introduces this chapter refers to a more recent study where four experienced cardiologists looked at 537 ECGs and were asked to tell whether the ECG pattern raised a suspicion of ischaemic heart disease. One or more cardiologists thought so in 20.3% of the cases, but all four agreed in only 3.7% of the cases.[31]

A statistical method, *kappa statistics*, has been developed which permits assessment of the reproducibility, i.e. the inter- or intra-observer agreement, independently of the accuracy.[37,38] I shall illustrate this method by means of a simple intra-observer study.

Sixty patients suspected of pulmonary embolism were subjected to pulmonary scintigraphy, and in 22 cases the scintigram was found to be positive.[39] Some months later, the scintigrams were re-read, and this time 14 were interpreted as positive. The results are shown in Table 2.2a, which reveals that 11 scintigrams were positive and 35 negative at both readings. Hence, the observed agreement was $(11 + 35)/60 = 0.77$ or 77%.

This measure of observer agreement is, however, quite misleading, as it does not take into account that the two readings will sometimes give the same result by chance. Imagine that the observer had not even looked at the scintigrams, but

Table 2.2 Inter-observer variation of pulmonary scintigraphy. a) Results of dual reading of 60 pulmonary scintigrams. b) Expected chance results if the diagnoses were mutually independent.

a)

		2nd Reading		
		Positive	Negative	Total
1st Reading	Positive	11	11	22
	Negative	3	35	38
	Total	14	46	60

b)

		2nd Reading		
		Positive	Negative	Total
1st Reading	Positive	5.13	16.87	22.00
	Negative	8.87	29.13	38.00
	Total	14.00	46.00	60.00

had simply selected some at random which he then said were positive. The first time he had selected 22 scintigrams and the second time 14. Then the frequency of positive findings would be 22/60 and 14/60, and the probability that a scintigram would be labelled positive both times would be $22/60 \times 14/60$. Consequently, as there were 60 patients, we should expect that $22/60 \times 14/60 \times 60$ scintigrams $= 5.13$ scintigrams would be labelled positive at both readings simply by chance. Similarly, it would be expected that $(38 \times 46)/60 = 29.13$ scintigrams would be labelled negative both times. These expected results are shown in Table 2.2b and we may conclude that the *expected rate of chance agreement* is $(5.13 + 29.13)/60 = 0.57$ or 57%. When this calculation is taken into account, the observed agreement rate of 77% is less impressive.

This approach to the problem has been formalized by the introduction of a statistic called κ (kappa) which relates the level of observed agreement to the level of chance agreement. In this case κ is 47% as the difference between observed agreement and chance agreement (77% − 57%) is only 47% of the

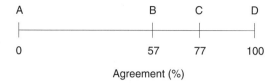

Fig. 2.2 Calculation of kappa. A: total disagreement, B: expected chance agreement, C: observed agreement, D: perfect agreement. The percentages refer to the example shown in Table 2.2.

difference between perfect agreement and chance agreement (100% − 57%). This idea is best explained by marking the agreement rates on a line as shown in Fig. 2.2. On this line the observed agreement rate (Point C) is situated 77% of the way from total disagreement (Point A) to perfect agreement (Point D), but it is only situated 47% of the way from expected chance agreement (Point B) to perfect agreement D).

The formal definition of kappa is:

$$\kappa = \frac{p_o - p_c}{1 - p_c}$$

where p_o is the observed and p_c is the expected chance agreement.

In principle, kappa may vary between −1 and 1. Kappa is 1 if the agreement is perfect; it is positive if the agreement is less than perfect, but larger than that expected by chance; and it is 0 if the agreement equals expected chance agreement. A negative kappa value makes little sense, as it suggests a systematic disagreement between the observers.

Kappa calculations present statistical problems,[40,41] but are helpful when clinicians wish to assess the reproducibility of the results of diagnostic tests. They provide no information about the accuracy of the test results, which must be assessed by means of the methods explained in Chapter 4.

The scintigraphy study is an example of an intra-observer study. It would have been an inter-observer study if two observers had assessed the same photos, but the calculations would have been just the same. Many such studies have been conducted,[42] and frequently the agreement is smaller than expected. In one study of the inter-observer agreement for gastroscopy, for instance, the kappa values were 0.59 for the diagnosis of gastric ulcers and 0.54 for the diagnosis of duodenal ulcers.[43,44] These results surprise gastroenterologists who believe that their observations are much more reliable.

Descriptive physical signs

The reproducibility of the observations that we make on the daily wardround is generally quite low, as it is often seen that doctors who examine the same patient disagree. That liver that was felt 3 cm below the costal margin on the Monday might no longer be palpable on the Tuesday, but perhaps a small goitre is found instead that was not demonstrated the day before.

In a study that assessed the reproducibility of clinical signs when doctors examine their patients' chests by auscultation and percussion, each of 202 newly admitted patients in a medical ward was examined by two doctors selected at random from all members of the medical staff.[45] The kappa values, which are shown in Table 2.3, were far from impressive, considering the fact that the doctors knew that they participated in a scientific study and probably did their best. Before the results were disclosed the doctors were asked to guess what the agreement would be like. This was done indirectly by means of numerical examples, which permitted the calculation of an expected kappa value. The average expected kappa values are shown in Table 2.3 in brackets and it is quite clear that the actual results did not fulfil the expectations. In this way the study illustrates that clinicians tend to overestimate substantially the reliability of their observations.

The accuracy of clinical signs can only be assessed if it is possible to determine the truth by some other method. When clinicians inspect the patient's conjunctiva they sometimes state that the patient is anaemic, and when they palpate the abdomen they may make a diagnosis of ascites. In such cases it is possible to assess the accuracy by determining the haemoglobin concentration of the blood or by doing an ultrasound scan of the abdomen, and it has been shown that very often the clinical diagnoses are wrong.[46,47]. In general, it is

Table 2.3 Inter-observer agreement for chest examination (auscultation and percussion). Selected results. The table shows the achieved kappa values and in brackets the expected kappa values.

Rhonchi	0.55	(0.82)
Fine moist sounds	0.36	(0.65)
Coarse moist sounds	0.15	(0.87)
Diminution of breath sounds	0.16	(0.75)
Prolonged expiration	0.53	(0.86)
Dullness	0.34	(0.79)

best to avoid diagnostic data transformation altogether, and to record only what was actually observed, e.g. paleness of the conjunctiva or a swollen abdomen (with perhaps absence of liver dullness). These clinical signs may not be reliable for diagnostic purposes, but they are still important as they suggest further investigations.

There are many reasons for the low reproducibility of some descriptive paraclinical and clinical data. Experience and thoroughness are important, but even experienced observers may disagree about definitions, or about the threshold of normality when there is a gradual transition between the normal and the abnormal. It is often possible to reduce the variation, however. The doctors who studied the reliability of pulmonary scintigraphy (as reported above) reached higher agreement when they repeated the study, after having standardized their descriptions.

Further, the examination will be more thorough and the threshold for recording a physical sign as abnormal will be lower if the diagnosis is already expected. I have mentioned earlier that radiologists may be biased by the information on the request form, and a physician doing a physical examination will be influenced by his knowledge of the patient's clinical picture. This risk of bias is inherent in clinical practice, but awareness of the problem may prevent the decision process from going astray.

The statistical concept of normality

The sum of the normal and abnormal clinical data that have been collected by the clinician constitute the patient's clinical picture, and all this information serves a variety of purposes. It may be used to decide whether or not the patient is ill, or it may help to confirm or exclude different diagnoses. It may also be used to assess the severity of the patient's condition, to monitor the course of the disease and to assess the treatment result. But before we discuss the relevance of clinical data for these purposes, it is necessary to consider the concept of normality and the concept of disease.

Doctors discussing their patients often use expressions such as 'the eosinophil count is high', 'the serum potassium is low', or 'the aminotransferase is normal'. These expressions illustrate that clinicians often reduce the scale of measurement from an interval scale to an ordinal scale, confining themselves to a distinction between abnormally low, normal and abnormally high values. They sometimes even use special terms to designate these categories, e.g. hypokalaemia, eosinophilia, hypertension, fever, thrombocytopenia and hypercholesterolaemia. All such expressions presuppose that we know what is normal, and in the case of chemical analyses we usually rely on the list of normal ranges that is issued by the local laboratory. Ideally, these normal ranges comprise 95% of the healthy population, which means that we shall expect every twentieth healthy person to present a value that is either 'abnormally' high or low.

Imagine a chemical pathologist, who wishes to determine the normal range for a new quantitative blood analysis and records the results in a sample of normal people. The distribution of the results can be visualized by a histogram, like the one shown in Fig. 2.3f, and, if the sample is sufficiently large, it may be possible to assess the shape of the distribution. It may, for instance, be positively skew (Fig. 2.3a), negatively skew (Fig. 2.3b) or bimodal (Fig. 2.3c). The distribution of the serum bilirubin is positively skew whereas the distribution of the serum concentration of a drug after ingestion of a fixed dose may be bimodal due to a mixture of slow and fast drug metabolizers. No prior assumptions are warranted as regards the shape and mathematical formula of the distribution,

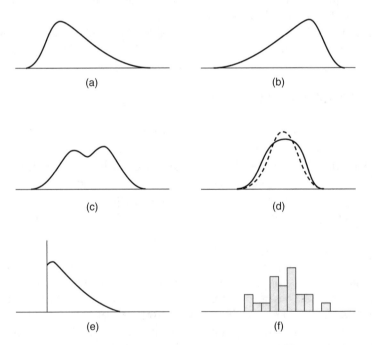

Fig. 2.3   Different types of distributions. a) Positively skew. b) Negatively skew. c) Bimodal. d) Bell shaped but non-Gaussian (the stippled curve is Gaussian). e) Truncated. f) Histogram of results from a small number of experiments.

and therefore the 95% interval cannot be calculated mathematically. Instead, one must rank all the observations in ascending order and cut off 2.5% of the results from each end. If, for instance, 200 normal people have been examined, the lowest five and the highest five results are removed, and the range of the remaining 190 results represents the *observed 95% range.* In statistical terminology the cut-off points are called the 2.5 and the 97.5 percentiles.

Previously, chemical pathologists did not always calculate the normal range in this way. Instead they calculated the standard deviation, as they assumed that mean ± two standard deviations might serve as the normal range. This calculation can often be used to assess the reproducibility of an analysis, as there is reason to believe that repeated measurements of the same sample will form a Gaussian distribution, but the Gaussian assumption may be unwarranted when we are dealing with single measurements from a large number of individuals. As noted previously, the Gaussian distribution is often called the normal distribution, but that may lead to misunderstandings, as, normally, many biological distributions are non-Gaussian.

Even bell-shaped and symmetric distributions need not be Gaussian as the Gaussian equation (Fig. 2.1) only fits one particular bell shape, and if we calculate mean ± two standard deviations for the bell-shaped, but non-Gaussian curve in Fig. 2.3d, the interval will not correspond to 95% of the area.

Today chemical pathologists are well aware of this problem, but others who report the distribution of some quantitative variable in a group of healthy people or patients have not yet learnt the lesson. Even the best medical journals publish numerous papers where the authors quote the mean and standard deviation of their results when this calculation is nonsensical. Once, for example, it was stated in a paper that the mean basic gastric acid output in gastric ulcer patients was 1.5 mmol H^+/hour and that the standard deviation was 2.4 mmol H^+/hour.[48] This must give the reader the impression that 95% of the patients produced between −3.3 and +6.3 mmol H^+/hour or, in other words, that some patients produced a base instead of an acid. The truth is, of course, that the distribution is truncated as shown in Fig. 2.3e.

This criticism of the standard deviation, however, only concerns its use for descriptive purposes. If the sample is large and the distribution not too skew, it may still be used to calculate the so-called standard error of the mean. The purpose of that calculation will be discussed in Chapter 8.

It is reasonable that clinicians often refer to the normal range, when they decide on the normality of a test result, but they should keep in mind how it was determined. They should remember that it is a 95% range and that, even in healthy people, one must expect every twentieth test result to be either too high or too low. If a healthy person is subjected to 20 blood tests (whose results are mutually independent) the probability of one or more abnormal results will be $1 - 0.95^{20} = 0.64$ or 64%. If normality is defined by the normal range, 'a normal person is anyone who has not been sufficiently investigated'.[6]

In other cases the relevance of the reference population is questionable. Is it, for instance, reasonable to use a normal range based on blood samples from blood donors or medical students when we decide on the normality of the serum albumin of a 75-year-old woman? Perhaps we ought to calculate a special normal range for the elderly. Bone mineral density, for instance, declines with age, and it is therefore not reasonable to define a normal value as that which is seen in a 30-year-old woman, as was once done.[49]

The concept of disease

The concepts of normality and abnormality cannot be fully explained by statistical considerations. They are closely related to the concepts of health and disease, as illustrated by the fact that we talk about normal health and as we regard disease as something abnormal. According to the statistical approach, normality is defined as that which is common, and this definition ignores the fact that sometimes disease is common and health rare. Once, for instance, it was normal (common) in Switzerland and some parts of the Balkans to suffer from hypothyroidism due to iodine deficiency, and in many parts of the world today it is normal (common) for children to be malnourished. Therefore, it is necessary to consider definitions of health and disease that do not depend on the statistical concept of normality. This is a central problem in medical philosophy,[13] but for the purpose of this book it is sufficient to present, very briefly, two opposing views.

According to one school of thought, health and disease are regarded as purely biological phenomena. It is taken to be an objective fact that a person is ill, as disease is regarded as a deviation from normal biological functioning, and in this context normal functioning does not mean that which is common, but that which a biological organism needs in order to thrive, reproduce and sustain life. Therefore, a patient with a pyloric stenosis is objectively ill, as he cannot thrive biologically unless the passage of food from the stomach into the gut is restored. This biological or objectivist concept of disease may well appeal to scientifically minded doctors, but it is obviously unsatisfactory from the point of view that it ignores that sick people 'feel ill' and suffer unpleasant subjective symptoms.

Therefore, other medical philosophers deny that the concept of disease can be reduced to an objective phenomenon. They adopt a subjectivist view of disease and maintain that the primary characteristics of the state of disease are the patient's feelings. This view, however, is also unsatisfactory, as the presence of unpleasant symptoms is not tantamount to being ill. We do not, for instance, say that a woman in labour is ill, but we regard the unconscious person or the person with an asymptomatic lung cancer as seriously ill.

The issue is further complicated by the influence of cultural norms. Once run-away slaves in the western hemisphere were thought to suffer from a special disease called drapetomania (from Greek *drapetes* = fugitive) and Russians who opposed Stalin were regarded as mentally ill and confined to psychiatric institutions. Now we no longer accept these 'diagnoses', just as we no longer regard homosexuality as a disease entity, but instead the 'hyperactivity' of some children and 'chronic fatigue syndrome' have found their place in the disease classification.

The threshold of iatrotropy also, to some extent, depends on social norms, and it is possible that some of those people who seek medical advice because of mild back pain or irritable bowel syndrome would previously have seen their recurring symptoms as an expression of the inescapable vicissitudes of life. Nowadays, a treatment is commonly instituted, e.g. for irritable bowel syndrome, even though the treatment, in some cases, can be deadly.[49,50]

The risk of *somatization* may also be mentioned in this context. Personal worries of any kind may lower the threshold of iatrotropy, and the visit to the doctor may lead to somatic diagnoses. In such cases the net result may well be that the patient's situation has become even more complicated than it was. The personal problems are not brought to light, and the somatic diagnosis causes new worries or even serves to legitimate the role as a patient and the institution of treatment.

It has become fashionable to propose the adoption of a *bio-psycho-social disease concept*, which serves to remind us that the disease concept has at least these three dimensions, and that it has proved impossible to define health and disease in simple terms. Clinicians must concern themselves with all aspects of the disease concept, and they must, in particular, take care that they do not pay so much attention to the biological aspect that they forget the others.

Some years ago, well-meaning Danish doctors placed themselves near the cash registers in supermarkets and offered to measure the customers' blood pressure, and those who were found to have an abnormal blood pressure were referred to their general practitioner. These doctors may have done some good, as it is possible that they detected some cases of hypertension which, years ahead, would have led to a cerebrovascular accident which was now averted, but the cost must not be overlooked. Some people might simply take it in their stride that from then on they had to take tablets and see their general practitioner at regular intervals, but others would start worrying about their state of health and the harmful effects of the drugs. They would feel that they were 'made ill' that day in the supermarket.

Regular 'health check-ups' which do not aim at detecting any particular disease are not as popular in Europe as in the United States, and it is doubtful whether they are ever warranted. A seemingly innocent health check-up may, for instance, entail a digital rectal exploration, and perhaps the doctor finds an enlarged prostate and asks for determination of the blood level of prostate specific antigen on suspicion of prostate cancer. This antigen is often increased in healthy, middle-aged men, but increased values lead to biopsies, and the microscopy will often reveal cancer lesions as such lesions are common.[51] The healthy male has now become a cancer patient and might get his prostate removed, which most often leads to permanent impotence.[52]

Mass screening for non-iatrotropic cases of particular diseases is, of course, sometimes fully justified, but nevertheless this activity contrasts with the classical role of the physician, which is to help those people who turn to him for help. It is a different thing altogether to approach people who live their lives believing that they are healthy, and then tell them that their good health is an illusion. It is particularly important to discuss this problem at a time when genetic screening has become a realistic possibility. There is a small chance that a disease responsive to treatment will be detected at an early stage, but there is also considerable risk that the 'check-up' leads to unnecessary worries due to false positive results or to truly abnormal results, which one cannot do anything about.

We also need to consider carefully the more permanent harm of mass screening, in particular of cancer screening. The vast majority of middle-aged people, or perhaps even everybody if they are examined enough, have cancerous lesions in one or more organs, which either disappear again or grow so slowly that they are essentially harmless since they do not give any symptoms before the persons die from other causes.[51] Usually, all such cancerous lesions are treated because, at present, we cannot determine in the microscope or otherwise which lesions are dangerous and which are harmless. Screening for cancer therefore makes many healthy citizens ill. Most often, many more people suffer the consequences of this overdiagnosis and overtreatment than those few who benefit from the screening.[51,53,54] Even more people, for some cancers about half of those screened,[51,54] will get a false positive diagnosis which can create much distress[55] that sometimes continues after they have been told it was a false alarm. It is also worth noting that so-called 'epidemics' of cancer have often been caused merely by increased diagnostic awareness and testing, resulting in the addition of many harmless cases and cases where the diagnosis is false (because the microscopic diagnosis is not particularly reliable), even for such feared diagnoses as malignant melanoma.[51]

Similarly, 'epidemics' of allergies may be nothing more than increased awareness and diagnosis of people with very mild symptoms who were previously undiagnosed. When we read about such results in the news, which routinely lead journalists to call for immediate political action, we must ask whether there has also been an increase in asthma (or even better, serious cases requiring hospital admission that will always be registered). Quite often, we will discover that this was not the case and that the 'epidemic' was probably artificial.

The drug industry has a major role in inventing new 'diseases' and in promoting diseases,[49,56] as it has a commercial interest in increasing the consumption of medicines in the population as much as possible. There can be little doubt that effective marketing is the main reason for the widespread, but mostly harmful, use of benzodiazepines and other tranquilizers and selective serotonin reuptake inhibitors against the worries of everyday life, and hormone replacement therapy for treatment of mild menopausal symptoms.

Interpretation and relevance

The development of clinical medicine is best appreciated by looking through old medical records. In the late 1920s the following paraclinical investigations, including routine tests, were carried out at a Danish hospital on a patient who was admitted suffering from severe diarrhoea and anaemia:

> Haemoglobin, colour index, WBC, differential count, Wassermann reaction, benzidine and catalase tests on stools, chest X-ray, barium meal (with follow-through to the colon), and urine microscopy and analysis for proteinuria.

Nowadays a patient admitted for the same reason might easily go through the following programme:

> Blood: ESR, haemoglobin, RBC, WBC, differential count, reticulocyte count, MCV, MCHC, C-reactive protein, erythrocyte folate. Serum: iron and iron-binding capacity, B_{12}, calcium, phosphate, magnesium, sodium, potassium, bicarbonate, albumin, creatinine, aminotransferase, alkaline phosphatase, bilirubin, coagulation factors, TSH and transglutaminase antibodies. Stools: blood, pathogenic bacteria, fat content, worms, eggs and cysts. Urine:

protein, glucose, nitrite and leucocytes. Coloscopy with biopsy, gastroscopy with jejunal biopsy, X-ray of small gut, ultrasound scan of the abdomen and lactose tolerance test. The results of these investigations may then lead to others, such as: pancreatic function tests, culture of duodenal aspirate and capsule endoscopy.

I do not necessarily imply that any of these investigations are superfluous, but, nevertheless, this example, and numerous others from all spheres of clinical medicine, call for critical thought. We must ask ourselves if the tests which we request are necessary, if we interpret the results correctly, and if they serve the purpose that we expect them to serve.

Probably, some of the tests that we do are not really required. It is customary, for instance, at many hospitals to check routinely the electrolyte status of all newly admitted patients and to measure their blood pressure at regular intervals during the first 24 hours. That may often be warranted, but in many cases we do not expect electrolyte disturbances or changes in the blood pressure, and then it might be more appropriate to give the patient the chance of a good rest.

Previously, it was also customary to do a routine chest X-ray and an ECG in all medical hospital patients, but in a survey of more than 400 patients with no history of cardiac or pulmonary disease the results did not influence the decision process.[57] According to a Swedish report, many routine investigations before planned operations have also been superfluous.[58] In a Dutch study, where the relevance of the tests requested by general practitioners was assessed every six months, the use of a number of common laboratory tests dropped by 38% over 10 years. In a different geographic area, which served as control, the number increased by 52% during the same period.[59]

Correct assessment of the results of quantitative laboratory tests requires an understanding of their reproducibility. Fig. 2.1a (p. 19) shows the random variation around the mean when we repeat the measurement of some substance in the same blood sample, and we shall, of course, expect similar variation when we do repeated tests on the same person over a period of time, even when the blood concentration is quite constant. If one day the laboratory returns a particularly high result, we shall, other things being equal, expect a lower result the next day, and vice versa. This phenomenon, which statisticians call *regression towards the mean*, is of considerable clinical interest. If, for instance, one abnormally high result prompts us to institute a particular treatment, we may well be led to believe that the normal result the next day indicates a treatment effect when, in fact, it only reflects the random variation of the results of the analysis. It is better to withhold treatment until we have repeated the test, but even that procedure is not foolproof. We must not, when we see an abnormally high result, repeat the test until the result falls within the normal range, and then conclude that the last result necessarily is the true one.

One must also keep in mind that the normal range only tells us whether or not a particular result is likely to occur in a population of healthy people, but that is not the real clinical problem. The clinician wants to know whether the test result is abnormal for that particular patient, and usually it is not possible to answer this question, except perhaps in retrospect. A patient with praecordial pain may have enzyme levels below the upper limit of the normal range, suggesting that he does not suffer from a myocardial infarction, but if the enzyme levels drop to the lower part of the normal range within a few days, it is reasonable to suspect that he had an infarction and that the results on admission were abnormally high in his case.

Indicators

The tests that we do serve different purposes and it might be possible to reduce the number of unnecessary investigations, if we always make it quite clear to ourselves why we request each individual test.

Firstly, clinical data may serve as *diagnostic indicators*, i.e. suggest different diagnostic possibilities. An elevated creatine kinase and certain ECG changes are diagnostic indicators of the disease myocardial infarction. The use of clinical data for this purpose will be discussed in Chapter 4.

Secondly, clinical data may be *prognostic indicators*, i.e. serve to predict the course of the disease. The prognosis of colonic cancer is relatively good if the histological examination shows that it is confined to the colonic mucosa, and it is poor if the cancer has spread to the regional lymph nodes. The NYHA, Apgar and APACHE scores are also used to assess the prognosis. Prognostic indicators that are used to predict the development of disease in healthy persons are often called risk factors.

Sometimes the situation is quite complex as the prognostic indicator may not be the direct cause of the good or bad outcome. It is well known, for instance, that the low mineral content of the bones in patients with osteoporosis predisposes to compression fractures, and, consequently, it was also thought that drugs that induce an increase in the mineral content would have a favourable effect on the prognosis. That, however, is not always true. Treatment with etidronate increases the mineral content and lowers the risk of fractures, but fluoride treatment increases the risk of fractures as well as the mineral content.[60] This example illustrates what is stressed throughout this book, that theoretical deductions should always be tested empirically.

Thirdly, clinical data are used as *clinical indicators* which means that they are used to assess the severity of the patient's condition at a given moment or to monitor the course of the disease. In everyday clinical practice repeated measurements of the body temperature are used to monitor the course of infectious diseases, and changes in blood pressure and pulse rate provide important information in cases of head trauma.

Patients with chronic diseases who are seen regularly in out-patient departments are, however, often subjected to investigations which are not well suited to monitor the course of the disease. Repeated X-ray examinations of the hands and feet and regular determinations of the erythrocyte sedimentation rate in patients with rheumatoid arthritis are good examples. The X-ray films can rarely be used to assess a treatment response as most available treatments have no effect on bone destructions, and the sedimentation rate is badly correlated to the extent of the inflammatory changes in the body. In these patients one may just as well rely on the clinical examination of the joints and the clinical impression of the patient's general condition.

Unnecessary investigations in patients with chronic diseases may even make matters worse. Patients with liver metastases and symptom-free HIV-positive people should be given the chance to live their lives as normally as possible, and repeated ultrasound scans or helper cell counts may enhance their awareness of the disease.

In general, clinicians pay greater attention to the results of paraclinical tests than to their own observations. The paraclinical results may be more objective and precise, especially if they represent interval scale measurements, but what is gained in reliability is easily lost in relevance as clinical decisions are usually based on judgments on an ordinal scale (this patient is very ill) and on a binary scale (should I continue to give this treatment?). These considerations are equally important for clinical research, especially for the planning of randomized clinical trials. I shall resume this discussion in Chapter 6.

3
The Disease Classification

'I seem to have an inflamed tongue, doctor. Will you have a look at it?'
'Ah, yes. You have got glossitis.'
'Thank you doctor. It's all right now I know what it is.'
Conversation quoted by Asher[61]

According to an old dictum 'there are no diseases, only sick people', and it is indisputably true that no two people with the same disease are exactly alike. Nonetheless, the disease classification is an indispensable tool in everyday clinical practice. The clinician who attempts to assess the patient's prognosis without treatment and with different forms of treatment makes use of the knowledge and experience which other clinicians before her have gained from the treatment of their patients. That knowledge and experience cannot, of course, be transmitted from one generation of doctors to the next in the form of thousands of case histories, but only as the collective experience with groups or classes of patients who resemble each other as regards disease mechanisms and clinical pictures. The disease classification represents such a classification of patients where each disease entity functions as a carrier of clinical knowledge.

This way of thinking is also well illustrated by the clinical decision process as it was sketched in Fig. 1.1 on p. 3. The clinician records the clinical picture of her patient, then she makes a diagnosis, which means that she finds out to which class of patients her patient belongs, and, finally, she exploits the collective experience which has been gained by treating such patients in order to choose the best treatment for her particular patient.

In this way the disease classification may be regarded as a nominal scale with a large number of classes, but unfortunately it is not that simple. Ideally, a nominal scale is exhaustive and exclusive, but the disease classification fulfils neither of these conditions. The contemporary classification, which constitutes the backbone of any textbook of clinical medicine, reflects the different ways of thinking of successive generations of medical doctors, and it is not logically satisfactory. Sometimes we see patients who cannot be referred to a recognized disease entity and sometimes a patient can be referred to several disease entities. The same patient may, for instance be said to suffer from chronic pancreatitis or from diabetes mellitus.

The historical perspective

A brief historical account of the development of the disease classification and the changing patterns of medical thinking[1,62] will make it easier to understand some of the complexities of clinical reasoning today.

The seventeenth and eighteenth centuries

In the seventeenth century, university teaching of medicine consisted of lectures, held in Latin, on Galenic, iatrochemical or some other dogmatic medical theory. However, the empiricist approach to science with its emphasis on observation and experimentation gradually gained ground. Thomas Sydenham (1624–84) is rightly regarded as one of the pioneers. He was a friend of the empiricist philosopher (and physician) John Locke and set out to describe, as objectively as possible, the clinical picture and the natural history of a number of diseases.

The following description of an attack of gout which is quoted from the English translation[62] of his *Tractatus de podagra et hydrope* from 1683 shows his abilities as a writer:

> The victim goes to bed and sleeps in good health. About two o'clock in the morning he is awakened by a severe pain in the great toe: more rarely in the heel, ankle or instep. This pain is like that of a dislocation, and yet the parts feel as if cold water were poured over them. Then follows chills and shivers and a little fever. The pain, which was at first moderate, becomes more intense ... Now it is a violent stretching and tearing of the ligaments – now it is a gnawing pain and now a pressure and tightening. So exquisite and lively meanwhile is the feeling of the

part affected, that it cannot bear the weight of the bedclothes ... the
night is passed in torture, sleeplessness, turning of the part affected,
and perpetual change of posture.

This description is perhaps particularly vivid as Sydenham himself suffered
from gout. Sydenham was the first to distinguish between scarlet fever and
measles and he also succeeded in making a distinction between chorea minor
and hysteria. He studied a number of the common epidemic diseases of his
time, including the Great Plague, which swept London in 1665 and in which
more than 50 000 people died.

The need for careful observations became more widely accepted in the eighteenth century. At that time the sum of knowledge in the natural sciences was
so limited that many scientists were still polymaths. Botanical taxonomy was
en vogue and, as many botanists were also physicians, attempts were made to
classify diseases like plants. François Boissier de Sauvages in Montpellier (1706–
67) wrote *Nosologia methodica* which subdivides 'diseases' into 10 classes, 295
genera and 2400 species, and the greatest of botanical taxonomists, Carolus
Linnæus (1707–78) composed a *Genera morborum*.

These early phases of the development of the disease classification are not
only of historical interest. The careful descriptions of different diseases that
we find in our textbooks follow the tradition from the time of Sydenham and
the taxonomists, and we still use symptom diagnoses and establish clinical
syndromes, if we have little knowledge of the causes and mechanisms of the
disease entity in question.

The empiricist approach, however, did not displace the old ways of thinking.
As late as the first half of the nineteenth century many physicians still accepted
the ancient doctrines of humoral pathology, according to which disease represents an imbalance of the four humours (yellow and black biles, blood and
phlegm), and other equally speculative systems of thought also reached considerable popularity. William Cullen (1712–90) believed that life is a function
of nervous energy and that diseases are mainly nervous disorders. Gout, for
instance, was classified as a neurosis. Clinicians may still, unconsciously, be
harking back to Cullen when they refer to a disease of unknown aetiology as
'probably nervous'.[62]

All the speculative theories from those days may be labelled pre- or pseudoscientific, as no attempt was made to test them empirically, but pseudoscientific thinking is by no means a thing of the past. The theoretical basis of
homoeopathy, reflexology and almost all other forms of so-called alternative
(or complementary) medicine are as speculative and empirically ill-founded
as Greek humoral pathology (see Chapter 5).

The nineteenth and twentieth centuries

At the beginning of the nineteenth century a new epoch in medical science was inaugurated. Xavier Bichat (1771–1802) published his *Anatomie générale* and during the following decades the French anatomists systematically described the anatomical lesions that they observed on the autopsy table. However, as illustrated by the work done by René Laënnec (1781–1826), their studies always served a clinical purpose. Laënnec was both a pathologist and a physician and as mentioned previously he introduced chest auscultation and correlated the auscultatory signs to anatomical lesions found at autopsy. He was particularly interested in tuberculosis and was the first to regard this disease as an entity. It had previously been split up into a number of 'diseases' according to the varied clinical manifestations. The ideas of the French anatomists spread to other centres, including Dublin (Graves, Stokes, Cheyne, Adams and Corrigan) and Guy's Hospital, London (Addison, Bright and Hodgkin). All these names are still remembered as eponyms.

This period of the history of medicine has left its stamp on our disease classification as the majority of diseases are still named after anatomical lesions. We are now so familiar with the tradition that was established in the early nineteenth century that it is difficult for us to appreciate to which extent it represented a radically new way of thinking. The taxonomists of that century had not distinguished between the patient's disease and the patient's clinical picture, but from the time of the French anatomists diseases were regarded as something localized inside the body. Physicians, of course, still paid attention to their patients' subjective symptoms, but from then on they saw it as their task to explain the symptoms by the demonstration of an anatomical lesion, i.e. an objective, abnormal finding. Objectivity became the hallmark of scientific medicine.

From the middle of the century it was no longer considered sufficient to describe the clinical and anatomical manifestations of disease. Physicians began to take an interest in the functions of the human organism. Rudolf Virchow (1821–1902), the founder of cellular pathology, gave pathological anatomy a dynamic dimension; he studied tumour growth, explained thromboembolism and was the first to observe leucocytosis. At that time a number of physiological journals were started in Germany and France, and Claude Bernard (1813–78) made great advances in physiology by means of carefully planned animal experiments. He showed in the 1850s that the liver contains glycogen and that pancreatic juice decomposes fat, starch and protein. He also studied the vasomotor mechanism and isolated vasodilator and vasoconstrictor nerves. The interest in experimental physiology led to the establishment of hospital laboratories, where clinicians could carry out paraclinical investigations on their patients and where they could do experimental research. This development has continued to our time and it has led to further specialization and the establishment of disciplines such as endocrinology and immunology. It has also left its stamp on the disease classification. Hypertension, renal failure, diabetes mellitus and thyrotoxicosis are but a few examples of conditions that today are defined in terms of a physiological or a metabolic dysfunction.

The introduction of laboratory research also led to the verification of the germ theory and the development of bacteriology, the pioneers being Louis Pasteur (1822–95) and Robert Koch (1843–1910). A variety of bacteria were discovered, and it became possible to classify diseases according to the infective agent. Typhoid fever, tuberculosis, malaria and measles are examples of diseases that today are defined by their bacterial, parasitic or viral aetiology. The development of microbiology also cemented the concept of 'one cause – one disease', which, among others, even Sydenham had advocated.

During the second half of the twentieth century we have seen the development of molecular biology as a very important new discipline. The molecules in question are primarily DNA and RNA and the demonstration of changes in the genome will undoubtedly leave its imprint on the disease classification in the years to come. It has been established already that many congenital diseases (often rare metabolic diseases) are caused by changes in a single gene, but numerous other diseases seem to be associated with mutations in several genes. Mutations that occur later in life may also lead to disease, e.g. cancer. This knowledge may have therapeutic consequences. Chronic myeloid leukaemia, for example, can be treated with a drug that abolishes the effect of a very active signalling protein.

From a philosophical point of view this presentation reflects what has been called the nominalistic concept of disease,[6] according to which the disease name denotes a class of patients who have something in common, e.g. an anatomical lesion or a functional disturbance. That is what is meant by the expression 'There are no diseases, only sick people'.

The justification of this point of view may seem self-evident, but nonetheless we often talk about diseases as if we accepted the essentialistic concept of disease, i.e. as if diseases had an independent existence. We say that diseases attack people and we describe their clinical manifestations almost as if they were demons, but we must regard such expressions as mere figures of speech. They must not make us forget that the disease classification is no more than a tool that reflects successive traditions of medical thinking. We gradually gain more knowledge about the causes and mechanisms of disease, and consequently the disease classification must, from time to time, be revised and refined.

The theoretical perspective

The mechanical model of disease

Modern medical thinking originated in the nineteenth century, and as described above the focus of attention changed from one period to the next. First, our predecessors only saw the structural changes (anatomical lesions) in the body and later on they paid more attention to functional (physiological or metabolic) disturbances, but basically their way of thinking did not change. The fruitful idea that gained ground two hundred years ago was the so-called mechanical model of disease, according to which man is seen as a complex 'machine' and disease as a fault in the machinery.

Of course, our predecessors did not overlook the importance of environmental or hereditary factors as determinants of disease. Since prehistoric times it has been known that poisonous berries may cause illness and it was understood, even prior to the discovery of bacteria, that disease may be passed from one person to another. It was also well known that some diseases, such as haemophilia, might run in families. According to the traditional mechanical model, the aetiological (environmental or hereditary) factors elicit the disease process that causes the fault in the machine.

Even today much medical thinking, both at the bedside and in the research laboratory, accords well with this interpretation of the mechanical model. Often, however, it is too simple, and then it may be more appropriate to regard the human organism as a self-regulating system. The organism seeks, much like a thermostat, to keep the body temperature at a constant level, by transpiration when it begins to rise and by shivering when it threatens to fall; it also tends to maintain the concentration of different hormones within narrow limits, and to regulate the blood pressure. Almost all physiological mechanisms are characterized by complex feedback mechanisms that aim at maintaining the normal balance or homoeostasis. All this is well known, but it is worth noticing that this way of thinking leads to a more refined concept of disease. Now the state of disease is not just seen as the end-result of a causal chain, but as an abnormal equilibrium of a self-regulating system. The normal equilibrium is health, disease develops when the equilibrium is disturbed, and the self-regulation of the system has the effect that in most cases the normal balance is re-established, i.e. the patient is cured, without medical intervention.

This way of thinking may be regarded as an extension of the traditional mechanical model, but it has ancient roots. According to humoral pathology, disease is regarded as an imbalance of the four humours and the adherents of that theory saw it as their aim to restore the normal equilibrium by supporting what they called the healing power of nature (*vis medicatrix naturae*). Their theory was false, but fundamentally their way of thinking is not outmoded.

Molecular biology

The mechanical model of disease, however, has its limitations, as it does not take into account that the human organism is not just an extremely complex 'physico-chemical machine', but a 'living machine'. The mechanical model focuses on the normal or abnormal function of a 'machine' which already exists, but ignores the fact that the human 'machine' is a biological organism which begins its existence as a zygote, grows to its adult form, 're-creates' itself throughout life, until its begins to degenerate and finally dies. Disease may arise if any of these complex processes run astray.

It was molecular biology that opened the door to an understanding of these processes. We now know that special patterns of nucleotide sequences in the genome may cause serious congenital diseases or just predispose to the development of particular diseases later in life. But molecular biology may also help us to understand so-called acquired diseases. The mechanical models take the 'machine' for granted, and therefore it is not surprising that, until recently, medical science made little headway in its attempts to explain the development of malignant diseases and the degenerative diseases of old age. The cells of our body die and are replaced by others at short intervals, and these diseases are associated with the process of re-creation that takes place throughout life. Colonic cancer is explained by successive mutations in the cells of the gut, and the ageing process of all parts of the body may be seen as the successive slightly deficient replication of many kinds of cells. Anybody who reads medical journals will have noticed the explosive growth of papers on the mechanisms involved, but in most areas our knowledge is still superficial and limited.

In the years to come molecular biology will undoubtedly result in a much better understanding of disease processes, but it is possible that the break with traditional thinking will be much deeper. In this chapter I have used the term 'the mechanical model' which may sound rather simplistic, but from a philosophical point of view it is justified. Scientific thinking in general, including, for instance, physiological thinking, has been 'mechanical' in the sense that it is founded in the Newtonian picture of the world, i.e. a world governed by simple laws of nature. However, by the end of the twentieth century we have witnessed the development of new revolutionary ideas that may completely change our view of nature. Different terms are used, and, depending on the approach, one may talk about complexity theory, nonlinear dynamics, chaos theory, fractal theory or the theory of open self-organizing systems.[63,64] Fractal geometry seems to play an important role in human morphogenesis.[64] A pattern is said to be fractal if it repeats itself on a smaller and smaller scale, and the finer and finer branches of arteries, bronchi and glandular ducts may be regarded as fractal-like structures.

In classical mechanics (linear dynamics) it is assumed that small changes of the initial values will only have small effects on the results. This, however, is not so when we are dealing with nonlinear physiological processes associated with complex feedback mechanisms where gradual small changes in the initial values may have striking and unanticipated effects. In studies of isolated muscle strips it was found, for instance, that a gradual increase in the intracellular calcium concentration provoked a regular series of sudden changes in the cardiac rhythm.[65] Anybody who has seen a patient suddenly develop a life-threatening ventricular fibrillation will acknowledge that further theoretical studies of this kind may have considerable clinical implications. Chaos theory may also contribute to our understanding of physiological processes in areas such as endocrinology, neurophysiology and renal physiology.

Disease and the environment

Not so long ago, on a biological time scale, man lived as a hunter-gatherer. He was, from an evolutionary point of view, adapted to those living conditions, and since then he has not changed much genetically. His way of living has, however, undergone repeated radical changes and it is not surprising that new living conditions are associated with new diseases. Therefore, the development of disease may also be viewed from the perspective of evolutionary biology,[66] and often it may be regarded as maladaptation to the environment.

According to McKeown[67] the population density in the Stone Age was so small that diseases such as smallpox, measles and whooping cough could not have existed. They appeared by adaptation of animal pathogens when people moved together in larger numbers and established the first agricultural societies about 10 000 years ago. Later civilizations were associated with other diseases, and although it is difficult for us to 'diagnose' the diseases which are described by physicians in ancient Greece and Rome and during the Middle Ages, there can be no doubt that the diseases which they saw differed from the ones which we see today. Now we see the spreading of the so-called diseases of civilization, such as atheroclerosis, diabetes and hypertension to the developing world, where, at the same time, people suffer from infectious diseases unknown in more developed countries.

The variability of the disease pattern, even during a limited time span, is well illustrated by the history of peptic ulcer disease, i.e. gastric and duodenal ulcers in Northern Europe. In 1881, With, who was Professor of Clinical Medicine at The University Hospital of Copenhagen, published a book on gastric ulcers[68] in which he related a series of dramatic case histories. Most of the patients were young women aged 20–30 years who were admitted with haematemesis or perforation and peritonitis. Most of them died and the autopsy revealed a gastric ulcer. X-ray examination was not yet available, and therefore the diagnosis could only be made with certainty at the autopsy table. With, however, believed that the disease was common, because cardialgia 'is so widespread in the Nordic countries that few women aged 15–30 years, especially from the working classes, are spared...' According to With, cardialgia was a strong pain in the upper abdomen which often induced the patients to bend forward pressing the abdomen against the edge of a table or the back of a chair. During a period of four years, 339 such patients were admitted to his unit. One third presented with haematemesis, and they constituted about 10% of all admissions. Only one patient was found to have a duodenal ulcer and since autopsies at that time were thorough, it may be assumed that duodenal ulcers were rare. A number of those patients who were admitted and died had previously received the diagnosis of 'nervous cardialgia', 'hysteria' or 'mother-sickness' because the disease often hit young girls who had left home to go into domestic service. Also in those days doctors made the imputation of a nervous origin of the symptoms when they did not know what was wrong. Numerous similar cases were observed in Great Britain during the latter half of the nineteenth century. Country practitioners found perforated ulcers in young women, which 'swept away beautiful young creatures within a few hours', one of the most tragic experiences of their lives.[69]

Towards the end of the nineteenth century this disease of young women disappeared and no present-day clinician has ever seen such patients. Gastric ulcer disease is still seen, but now the disease occurs later in life in both men and women.

Then, at the beginning of the twentieth century, the presentation of 'peptic ulcer disease' took a new unexpected turn. As something quite new, numerous cases of duodenal ulcers were reported among young men. That clinical picture is still known, but it has changed throughout the century. Gradually, the patients' age at the onset of the disease has increased, and the disease is becoming less frequent.

We still do not know the environmental factors that caused the gastric ulcers in young women in the nineteenth century, but we know something about the aetiology of duodenal ulcer disease. It seems that the presence of Helicobacter pylori in the gastric mucosa is a necessary causal factor, and one can assume that this infection first appeared at the beginning of the nineteenth century. The prevalence of Helicobacter infection, which seems to be life long, has decreased throughout the century and today it is rare among younger people. We still do not know why so many young men were suddenly infected a hundred years ago and we do not know why it is not happening any longer. Now we can cure the disease with suitable antibiotic therapy, but probably duodenal ulcer disease would have disappeared spontaneously, even if the medical profession had never found the bacillus. It is a disease of the twentieth century.

The changing history of peptic ulcer disease is just one example of the dependence of the disease pattern on our living conditions. It should remind us that new, radical changes in our way of living are bound to lead to new infectious and non-infectious diseases. AIDS came as a big surprise not so many years ago, but our ever-changing environment will undoubtedly lead to other equally unexpected serious health problems in the years to come.

The practical perspective

The disease classification serves to organize all that knowledge and experience that has been assembled by studying individual patients, and that knowledge is then transmitted in a concise form through the publication of textbooks. The books are written within the traditions described above, and usually each disease has its own chapter, the heading of which is the disease name. The structure of the chapters may vary, but typically the information is organized as follows: definition, causes (aetiology and pathogenesis), clinical picture, prognosis, diagnosis and treatment.

Name of disease

Sometimes the name of the disease tells us which patients are described in that particular chapter, i.e. how the disease is defined. It is, for instance, obvious that a chapter entitled myocardial infarction deals with patients characterized by that particular anatomical lesion. But in many other cases it is difficult to interpret the disease name, or the name may refer to an obsolete definition of the disease.

The etymology of disease names provides interesting information about the history of medical thinking. Diabetes mellitus, for instance (from Greek 'passing through' and Latin 'honey-sweet') should remind us of the days when doctors tasted their patients' urine and distinguished between cases where the taste was sweet and those where it was 'insipid'. The disease name malaria reminds us that it was once thought that this type of fever was caused by *mal aria*, i.e. bad air, and in rheumatism, with its varying symptomatology, it was imagined that the causative agent flowed through the body (Greek *rheos* = flow or stream).

Definition

The disease name may be informative or of cultural interest, but usually it does not provide a satisfactory definition. As described above, the disease classification was created by generations of physicians belonging to different traditions, and textbook authors ought to define exactly which class of patients is described in each chapter. In other words, they ought to fix a set of criteria which are fulfilled by all patients who are said to have the disease and which are not fulfilled by those who are said not to have the disease.

Usually, however, this is not done. Often textbook authors provide no definition at all, or they include what they call a 'definition', which on closer inspection is only an ultrashort description. This deficiency would be of little practical significance, if there was consensus among doctors when they make different diagnoses, but unfortunately this is not so, as illustrated by a classical example from psychiatry. American and British doctors often disagreed how to treat schizophrenia, as the Americans, in contrast to their British colleagues, found that psychotherapy was beneficial. This puzzle was solved when it was revealed that patients, who in Europe were said to have a neurosis, across the Atlantic were diagnosed as suffering from schizophrenia.[70] Somatic medicine offers similar examples. One might think that it would be easy to distinguish between gastric and duodenal ulcers, but there has been little agreement among gastroenterologists. Ulcers in the pyloric canal may be referred to either class, and some gastroenterologists have even held that all those ulcers that are located in the (ill-defined) prepyloric region of the stomach are 'really' duodenal ulcers.

The dearth of explicit, logically satisfactory definitions in the textbooks may have considerable practical consequences. The disease classification serves to organize clinical knowledge and experience, and a clinician cannot utilize the experience which another clinician has acquired treating patients with schizophrenia, duodenal ulcers, Crohn's disease, systemic lupus or numerous other diseases, if they do not use these diagnostic terms in the same way.

It is not easy, however, to define a disease entity. The problems are closely linked to the complexity of the disease classification, and it is necessary to distinguish between: symptom diagnoses, clinical syndromes, anatomically defined diseases, physiologically or metabolically defined diseases, and aetiologically defined diseases.

Symptom diagnoses

Symptom diagnoses that are based on the presence of a single symptom represent the most primitive form of disease entity. The diagnosis 'chronic diarrhoea' may serve as an example. The definition of this disease causes no problems, as the name indicates the defining criterion. The only requirement is that we have defined what we mean by the words 'diarrhoea' and 'chronic'. General practitioners frequently use this diagnosis when they refer one of their patients to a gastroenterologist in the hope that the specialist will be able to find the cause of the patient's symptom. If the subsequent examinations show that the patient suffers from a cancer of the colon (anatomical diagnosis), ulcerative colitis (syndrome) or lactase deficiency (metabolically defined disease), then the patient receives that diagnosis instead. Symptom diagnoses are subordinate to the other types of disease entities. Sometimes, however, the specialist is not able to make a more specific diagnosis and then the patient is referred back to the general practitioner with the unchanged diagnosis 'chronic diarrhoea'. This simple example shows that symptom diagnoses are used either as preliminary diagnoses or as diagnoses made by elimination. We disregard the possibility that the specialist will not admit her ignorance and pins the unsubstantiated diagnosis 'nervous diarrhoea' on her patient.

The name of a disease may sometimes suggest that our knowledge is greater than it is. As already discussed, the diagnosis of gastritis is sometimes used by clinicians when patients complain of upper abdominal pain for which no explanation can be found. This is a typical example of a symptom diagnosis made by elimination, but the primitive diagnosis has been disguised as an anatomically defined disease.

Syndromes

The general practitioner, Caleb Parry of Bath, described 'exophthalmic goitre' in 1786. Later the disease was also described by Graves (1835) in England,

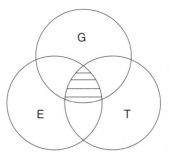

Fig. 3.1 The Merseburg triad. Patients with this syndrome are found in the hatched intersection of set G (patients with goitre), set E (patients with exophthalmus) and set T (patients with tachycardia).

and by Basedow (1840) in Germany, hence the designations Graves' disease in some countries and Basedow's disease in others. Carl August Basedow was a general practitioner in Merseburg and his description is the most interesting for our purpose, as he based the diagnosis on the simultaneous presence of three clinical signs: goitre, exophthalmus and tachycardia (the so-called Merseburg triad). The relationship is shown in the diagram in Fig. 3.1 where patients with 'Basedow's disease' are found in the intersection of the sets G, E and T. This triad is an example of a simple syndrome that is defined by the simultaneous presence of a fixed combination of clinical data. Later, when the function of the thyroid gland became known, this syndrome definition became obsolete, as 'Basedow's disease' was replaced by the metabolically defined disease entity, hyperthyroidism. Usually, however, disease entities defined on different levels do not delimit exactly the same patients, and that also holds true in this case. Many patients with hyperthyroidism do not fulfil Basedow's original criteria.

There are still many diseases where the pathogenesis is largely unknown, and then we still content ourselves with syndrome definitions. Ulcerative colitis is a good example. This disease name suggests that the disease entity can be defined histologically, but nevertheless pathologists will tell us that in many cases of that disease the histological picture is indistinguishable from that in other inflammatory diseases of the colon. If we make a list of all symptoms and signs found in patients who are diagnosed as having the disease, it will be found that no single symptom or sign, nor any simple combination of clinical data, fulfil the requirements of a defining criterion. However, we still have to accept the necessity of defining what is understood by this diagnosis, and therefore we must avail ourselves of a composite syndrome definition. Such a definition is illustrated by Fig. 3.2.[71] The set P comprises patients who present characteristic

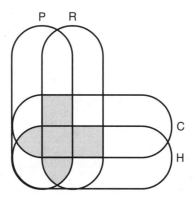

Fig. 3.2 Arbitrary syndrome definition of ulcerative colitis. The four sets comprise patients with characteristic sigmoidoscopic findings, i.e. proctitis (P), characteristic radiological findings (R), characteristic cytological or histological findings (C) and a characteristic history (H). The set of patients who present at least three of the four characteristics is indicated by the grey area.

sigmoidoscopic findings, i.e. patients with haemorrhagic proctitis; the set R comprises patients who present characteristic radiological findings; the set C comprises patients with characteristic histological and cytological findings (e.g. inflammatory cells in imprints of the rectal mucosa); and the set H comprises patients presenting a characteristic history (e.g. blood in the stools). In order to make the diagnosis it is required that three of these four criteria are fulfilled, which means that the patient must belong to one of the five grey subsets in Fig. 3.2.

In addition, it is required that no colonic cancer has been found which could explain the clinical picture, and that no aetiologically defined infectious disease (e.g. amoebic dysentery) has been demonstrated. Syndrome diagnoses are subordinate to anatomically defined and causally defined diseases.

This definition is not universally accepted, as clinicians elsewhere use different more or less well-defined criteria, but in some instances scientific societies have agreed on syndrome definitions in order to ensure consensus. As an example, the American Rheumatism Association[72] has proposed a syndrome definition of rheumatoid arthritis comprising the following criteria which are quoted in many textbooks:

1. Morning stiffness;

2. Arthritis in three or more joints;

3. Arthritis in hand joints;

4. Symmetric arthritis;

5. Subcutaneous nodules;

6. Positive reaction for rheumatoid factor;

7. Radiological changes in the joints.

Each of these criteria has been further defined, and a patient is said to suffer from rheumatoid arthritis if she fulfils at least four of these seven criteria. Other rheumatological diseases, such as systemic lupus erythematosus have been defined in a similar manner.

Anatomically defined diseases

As a legacy of medical thinking at the beginning of the nineteenth century many disease names designate anatomical lesions. Sometimes the designation is false (e.g. gastritis) or nonspecific (e.g. ulcerative colitis), but often the anatomical lesion serves well as the defining criterion. Rectal cancer, gastric ulcer, fracture of the neck of the femur and myocardial infarction are good examples.

From a practical point of view it is important in such cases to distinguish between two types of defining criteria. The criterion is said to be *accessible* if it is possible to ascertain, at the time of diagnosis, whether it is present or absent in a particular patient, and it is said to be *concealed* if this is not the case. A rectal cancer is accessible with proctoscopy, a gastric ulcer with gastroscopy and a hip fracture by looking at the X-ray picture. In contrast, it is not yet possible to ascertain by direct means whether or not a patient harbours a myocardial infarction, for which reason this defining criterion must be regarded as concealed.

If a disease is defined by a concealed criterion, it is necessary, for practical purposes, to supplement the theoretical definition with a *working definition*, in order to ensure maximum consensus as regards the use of the diagnostic term. Usually such working definitions take the form of a composite syndrome definition, like those mentioned above.

Some concealed criteria may be accessible in retrospect, i.e. they become accessible after the diagnostic situation. The presence of inflammation in the appendix is a concealed criterion when the diagnosis is made, but it becomes accessible when the surgeon performs a laparotomy. Similarly, the myocardial infarction becomes accessible, if the patient dies and an autopsy is made. Sometimes the anatomical defining criterion is accessible in some patients and concealed in others. It is, for instance, not always possible to prove or disprove that a patient suffers from a small pancreatic cancer.

This terminology is the key to the discussion about rational diagnosis that follows in Chapter 4.

Physiologically or metabolically defined diseases

This is a large heterogeneous group of diseases that are defined by our knowledge of the underlying physiological or metabolic malfunction. Sometimes the defining criterion is a single clinical or paraclinical finding, such as arterial hypertension or hypercholesterolaemia. The blood pressure and the cholesterol concentration are measured on an interval scale, and the definition of the disease depends on the rather arbitrary distinction between normal and abnormal levels.

In other cases it is much more difficult to define the disease. From a theoretical point of view it is, of course, uncontroversial to define hyperthyroidism as a disease caused by hyperfunction of the thyroid gland, diabetes mellitus as a particular disturbance of carbohydrate metabolism and bronchial asthma as bronchoconstriction mediated by an allergic reaction, but in practice these diagnoses are based on combinations of clinical data. Also in these cases we must rely on composite syndrome definitions.

Aetiologically defined diseases

This group of diseases comprises infectious diseases (e.g. typhoid fever), genetically defined, hereditary diseases (e.g. Huntington's chorea), poisonings and diseases defined by a particular environmental causal agent (e.g. asbestosis). Often the definitions combine aetiological and anatomical criteria, e.g. pneumococcal meningitis or renal tuberculosis.

Causes of disease (aetiology and pathogenesis)

According to the traditional mechanical model of disease, the clinical picture observed by the clinician is regarded as the end result of a causal chain (Fig. 3.3).

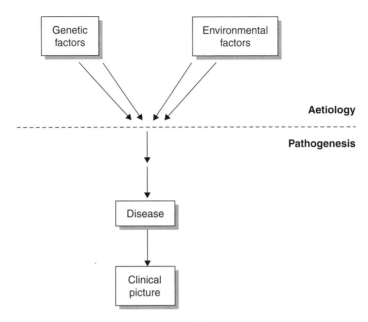

Fig. 3.3 The disease process.

The disease process is elicited by a combination of genetic and environmental factors that together constitute the *aetiology* (from Greek *aitia* = cause). Then follows a series of changes in the organism, which may be described in physiological, biochemical, immunological or morphological terms, and collectively these changes constitute the disease mechanism or *pathogenesis* of the disease (*pathos* = suffering and *genesis* = generation, creation). This causal chain results in the disease, i.e. 'mechanical fault' that causes the clinical picture. Textbooks frequently contain short sections on the aetiology and pathogenesis of various diseases, but usually no sharp distinction is made between the two terms.

In order to appreciate the complexity of the causation of disease, it is necessary to consider briefly the concept of causality. This is a difficult topic, but for our purpose it is permissible to ignore the philosophical implications[13] and to confine ourselves to a discussion of a few simple terms. In everyday language we often say that one event X is the cause of another event Y. This wording may give the impression that an event is always caused by another single event, and to avoid that misunderstanding it is better to state that the event X is one of the factors that determine event Y. When this terminology is used it is possible to distinguish between necessary, sufficient and contributory determinants.

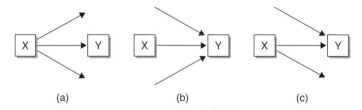

Fig. 3.4 Different types of causal relationships. a) X is a necessary determinant of Y, as Y is always preceded by X. b) X is a sufficient determinant of Y, as X is always succeeded by Y. c) X is a contributory determinant of Y, as X is sometimes succeeded by Y, and Y is sometimes preceded by X.

Factor X is a *necessary* determinant, if X always precedes Y, which of course does not imply that Y always succeeds X (Fig. 3.4a). We can illustrate this relationship by the determinant 'introduction into the organism of tubercle bacilli' and the effect 'pulmonary tuberculosis'. This disease is always preceded by the introduction of those bacilli, but the introduction of the bacilli does not always result in the disease. The reason for the great variation in the susceptibility of humans to infection is not fully established, but we cover up our ignorance by saying that the general resistance varies.

Pulmonary tuberculosis is a typical example of a disease about which it is often said that the aetiology is known, i.e. that *the* cause is known. It would be more correct to state that a single necessary determinant has been found, but even that information is of great practical importance. The progression of the disease depends on the continued presence of the necessary determinant, and therefore elimination of the determinant will halt the disease process. Unfortunately, however, this is not the case with all diseases. We also know one necessary determinant for the development of rheumatic fever (infection with haemolytic streptococci) but the therapeutic consequence of this knowledge is smaller, as the disease may progress in spite of the elimination of the aetiological determinant.

Factor X is a *sufficient* determinant, if X is always followed by Y (Fig. 3.4b), which of course does not imply that Y is always preceded by X. This causal relationship can be exemplified by the determinant 'lack of iron in the food' and the effect 'anaemia'. If the body is not supplied with iron over a period of time, then anaemia is always the result, but anaemia frequently has different causes. Knowledge of a sufficient determinant may also be used therapeutically, but it is less useful from a clinical point of view. Treatment of an anaemic patient with iron will only be effective if iron deficiency is a determining factor in that particular patient. For this reason 'anaemia' is not considered a satisfactory disease entity, and it is subdivided into smaller entities, like iron-deficiency or vitamin B_{12}-deficiency anaemia, each of which is characterized by a single necessary determinant.

Some determinants are neither necessary nor sufficient, but only contributory. This term is used if some factor X leads to an increased probability of Y, though X does not always lead to Y and Y is not always preceded by X (Fig. 3.4c). The logical status of contributory factors in the causal network may be difficult to define, but usually, the contributory factor is a necessary (but insufficient) component of a part of the causal complex in a subgroup of patients with a particular disease.[13,73] Arterial hypertension, for instance, is a contributory determinant of myocardial infarction as myocardial infarction is more frequent among hypertensives than among others, and that probably means that some patients with a myocardial infarction would not have developed the disease if they had not had hypertension. There are numerous other examples of contributory factors in medicine, e.g. familial predisposition to allergic diseases, increased acid production in duodenal ulcer disease and obesity in diabetes. Knowledge of contributory determinants may sometimes be used therapeutically, as illustrated by obese patients whose diabetes responds to weight loss.

The exploration of causal relationships in clinical medicine is difficult. Often a variety of causal factors interact, or the effects are modified by feedback mechanisms that serve to maintain normal homoeostasis. Therefore, it is not surprising that the results of clinical research are often misinterpreted. Suppose, for instance, that part of the population in a developing country was vaccinated before it was hit by an epidemic and that the vaccinated people were infected less frequently than the nonvaccinated ones. The most tempting conclusion is, of course, that the vaccination was effective (was a contributory determinant of the prevention of infection), but there are other possible explanations. Perhaps the offer to vaccinate was circulated in such a way that only those people who could read were vaccinated and that they lived under more hygienic conditions. Then, the relationship between vaccination and protection against infection might be due to a common cause (a *confounder*), the higher level of education (Fig. 3.5a). It is also possible that those who were vaccinated were told at

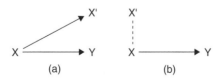

Fig. 3.5 Spurious causal relationships. a) X′ is not the cause of Y, but X′ and Y have a common cause. b) X′ is not the cause of Y, but is a concomitant factor to X.

the vaccination posts that they must boil all water, and that this precaution protected them against the epidemic. Then, the vaccination was a *concomitant factor* to the real determining factor, the boiling of drinking water (Fig. 3.5b). Finally, it is possible that the observed relationship between and protection against disease was a simple coincidence, i.e. that the low infection rate after vaccination was due to chance.

It may also be difficult to determine what is the cause and what is the effect. When it was first found that the prevalence of Helicobacter pylori infection among duodenal ulcer patients is very high, it was thought by some that it was a secondary phenomenon, but now it is known that the bacillus plays a causal role, probably as a necessary (but insufficient) determinant. The interpretation of a relationship between unemployment and alcoholism is also complicated. Alcoholism may lead to unemployment, unemployment may lead to alcoholism, the two factors may interact, or they may both be caused by psychological problems.

The reader of a textbook of medicine may easily get the impression that the causes of many diseases are well known, but when it is stated that the aetiology is known it usually only means that one of many aetiological factors has been isolated, and when it is stated that the pathogenesis is known, it usually only means that a few links in the chain of events leading to the observed clinical picture have been discovered. Medical scientists still find it difficult to abandon the time-honoured concept of one cause – one disease and to accept the idea of multiple determining factors. It is currently said about more and more diseases that they are 'genetic', and that may well be true in the limited sense that the genetic disposition is a contributory determinant. Usually, however, there are also environmental determinants, and it is easier to change the environment than to change the genome.

The clinical picture

The textbook describes the clinical pictures of those patients who are diagnosed as having different diseases. Thus, it will be stated in the chapter on myocardial infarction that the patients may present various symptoms (e.g. praecordial pain and anxiety), various clinical signs (tachycardia and sometimes a pericardial friction rub), and various paraclinical findings (e.g. certain electrocardiographic changes and changes in the blood concentration of different enzymes). The description of other diseases may include radiological and histological paraclinical findings such as a density on the chest X-ray in pneumonia and villous atrophy in gluten intolerance. All such clinical data are accessible, and it will often be mentioned whether they occur rarely, frequently or always in the disease in question. Other clinical data are concealed, e.g. an infarction in the mycocardium or the degeneration of the islets of Langerhans in diabetes.

The description of the disease is not limited to a listing of the symptoms and signs. The onset, progression, possible complications and short-term prognosis of the disease are also described. Most patients, however, also wish to know to what extent a newly diagnosed disease is likely to influence their future lives, and therefore it is unfortunate that often the textbooks provide less information about the long-term prognosis. The reason for this deficiency may well be that the textbooks are written by hospital specialists who in most cases refer their patients back to the general practitioner when the condition is stable and adequate treatment has been instituted. Some patients with chronic or recurring diseases will, of course, attend follow-up clinics at the hospital for a period of time, and others will be referred to hospital once again, if the disease takes an unexpected course, but on the whole the experience of hospital specialists, as regards the long-term prognosis of many diseases, is limited and biased. There is a great need for clinical research where unselected groups of patients with different diseases are followed for many years. Questions about the long-term prognosis of the individual patient can, of course, only be answered in probabilistic terms, but the predictions may be more precise if they are based on prospective studies where the outcome of the disease is correlated to the patients' clinical picture at the time of diagnosis. One may, for instance, draw diagrams, like the one shown for ulcerative colitis (Fig. 3.2), and determine the prognosis for each subset of patients.

As pointed out, the disease classification is a classification of patients. Each textbook chapter deals with a category of patients who are said to have a particular disease, and the reader who wishes to use that information must assume that her patients do not differ significantly from those described in the book. It cannot, however, be taken for granted that this assumption is fulfilled. The pattern of disease changes over time, due to our changing living conditions, and the classes of patients said to suffer from particular diseases also change due to the introduction of new diagnostic methods. Therefore, the textbooks must be rewritten from time to time, but unfortunately there is considerable inertia, and, probably, most textbooks describe the disease pattern 10 or more years before the date of publication.

Those who are diagnosed with a disease today are often considerably healthier than those who were diagnosed in previous decades. The introduction of more sensitive diagnostic methods, mass screening and health 'check-ups' all contribute to this development. Most important, however, are commercial pressures from the drug industry for lowering the threshold for what is considered normal. As a grotesque example of the latter, European guidelines on prevention of cardiovascular disease from 2003 defined hypertension and hypercholesterolaemia in such a way that 50% of Norwegian males 'suffer' from one or both of these 'diseases' from the age of 24,[74] although Norwegian males have one of the longest life expectancies in the world. Even a condition called 'prehypertension' has found its way into official guidelines.[49] Readers of such guidelines should know, however, that the specialists who write them often have undeclared financial conflicts of interest, having been paid by the drug companies for various services.[49]

Geographical variation also plays an important role. It cannot be taken for granted that, for instance, European patients resemble American patients in all respects, and there are obvious problems when doctors in developing countries consult textbooks describing patients in the industrialized world. But even within a particular society doctors must be careful when they consult their textbooks. Most textbooks are written by hospital specialists, and they do not see the same patients as general practitioners. They see different sections of the clinical spectrum.

The clinical spectrum

Arterial hypertension may serve as an example. This disease is not uncommon in hospital practice, but most patients with this diagnosis are examined and treated in general practice. In addition, there are numerous people who fulfil the definition of the disease by having high blood pressure, who do not seek medical advice, either because they suffer no symptoms at all or because they accept their mild symptoms. Then the hypertension will only be detected if the patients see their doctor for some other reason and the doctor routinely measures the blood pressure.

Thus, a disease like hypertension presents a clinical spectrum like the one shown in Fig. 3.6. The spectrum comprises three types of patients with the disease:

1. Non-iatrotropic cases, i.e. those cases where the patient does not seek medical advice either because she has no symptoms, or because the intensity of the symptoms has not reached the threshold of iatrotropy;

2. Iatrotropic cases that are seen by general practitioners;

3. Iatrotropic cases that have reached the hospitals.

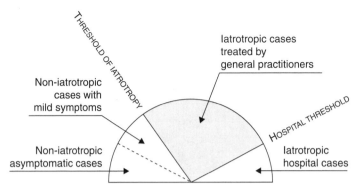

Fig. 3.6 The clinical spectrum.

Many diseases present such a spectrum and it is sometimes possible to distinguish between even more types of cases. In ulcerative colitis and Crohn's disease, for instance, one may also distinguish between those patients who are seen by medical gastroenterologists and those who are referred to a surgical department.

Most studies today are done at teaching hospitals, but they ought to be supplemented by clinical research in general practice, both diagnostic and prognostic studies, and randomized clinical trials.

Diagnosis and treatment

The textbook chapters on different diseases also contain information about diagnosis and treatment. The diagnostic process and the treatment decision will be discussed in detail in the following chapters, and here I shall only make one comment. There is an increasing awareness of the need for *evidence-based medicine* which implies that the efficacy of diagnostic tests and therapeutic interventions must be assessed by means of controlled clinical research. Standard textbooks provide more evidence-based information than before, but it is still common that the readers are not told anything about the rate of false positive and false negative results using different diagnostic tests, or about the therapeutic gain using different treatments. When the authors recommend different treatments they usually refer to the mechanism of action and not to the results of randomized clinical trials.

4
Diagnosis

The diagnostic problem of to-day has greatly changed
– the change has come to stay;
We all have to confess, though with a sigh
On complicated tests we much rely
And use too little hand and ear and eye.

Zeta[75]

The presentation of the diagnostic process in Chapter 1 was very brief. It was mentioned that the clinician examines his patient (collects clinical data) and then compares the patient's clinical picture with the manifestations of different diseases as they are described in the textbooks. In real life diagnostic reasoning is much more complex, and the following three patients demonstrate that it may vary from case to case.

A young man with jaundice is admitted to a teaching hospital. The consultant explains to the students that in order to make a diagnosis it is necessary to reason systematically. He tells them about the excretion of bilirubin and explains that jaundice may be caused by haemolysis, by liver-cell damage or by an occlusion of the common bile duct. He also explains which diseases may cause these disturbances and suggests what he calls a rational plan for the examination of the patient. This case illustrates the *deductive approach* to diagnosis as the clinician deduces from his pathophysiological knowledge what may be the cause of the symptom.

A middle-aged woman develops a burning pain in the left side of the chest. Inspection reveals a vesicular eruption stretching along the ribs from the spine to the sternum. The physician immediately recognizes this clinical picture and makes a diagnosis of herpes zoster. This diagnostic method may appropriately be called *pattern recognition*.

A young woman is admitted with fever and pain in the right iliac fossa associated with both direct and indirect tenderness. The surgeon knows that this clinical picture in all probability, but not with certainty, is caused by an acute appendicitis, and he decides to do a laparotomy. This is an example of *probabilistic diagnosis*.

These three types of diagnostic reasoning can, of course, rarely be isolated. The medical consultant, for instance, knew very well that haemolysis is a rare condition and that therefore this cause of jaundice is less probable than the others, and the surgeon recognized the pattern of an acute abdomen. The first part of this chapter will be devoted to probabilistic diagnosis, but later I shall consider pattern recognition and the strategy of bedside diagnosis.

The diagnostic universe

First, we shall consider the assessment of qualitative diagnostic tests, i.e. tests that provide results that are either positive or negative. The discussion of the reliability of such results requires that we distinguish between their reproducibility and their accuracy. It was explained in Chapter 2 that the reproducibility is assessed by means of inter-observer studies and calculation of kappa values, and here we shall only consider the accuracy of the test results. The assessment of accuracy presupposes that the true diagnosis is accessible and therefore we must make the very important assumption that it is possible to establish or exclude the diagnosis with certainty by means of an independent method.

From a clinical point of view, diagnostic tests serve two different purposes. They may be used to confirm that a patient suffers from a particular disease, or they may be used to exclude that this is the case, and usually the same test does not serve both purposes equally well. Confirmation of a diagnosis requires that the positive test results are reliable, whereas exclusion of a diagnosis requires that the negative results can be relied upon.

Microscopy of the sputum for the diagnosis of pulmonary tuberculosis is a good example of a test that provides reliable positive results. The discovery of an abundance of acid-fast bacilli in the sputum leaves little doubt that the patient suffers from this disease, but, of course, the absence of bacilli does not exclude the diagnosis. A simple chest X-ray, on the other hand, provides reliable negative results. Here the probability of pulmonary tuberculosis is minimal, if the films are completely normal, whereas the observation of a shadow in one

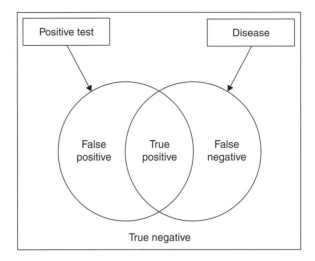

Fig. 4.1 The diagnostic universe.

of the lungs is less reliable from a diagnostic point of view, as it is often difficult to distinguish between tuberculous infiltrations and infiltrations caused by pneumonia or lung cancer.

In most cases, however, neither the positive nor the negative test results are fully reliable. This situation may be illustrated by a simple diagram (Fig. 4.1) where the rectangle represents the diagnostic universe, i.e. all patients presenting a particular clinical picture. Some of the patients have a particular disease (the circle to the right) and some present a positive result of the diagnostic test (the circle to the left). These two sets of patients overlap, dividing the universe into four subsets which represent patients with true positive results (those with a positive test who have the disease), false positive results (those with a positive test who do not have the disease), true negative results (those with a negative test who do not have the disease) and false negative results (those with a negative test who have the disease).

In order to assess the accuracy of the test results we must determine the number of patients in each subset, and these numbers may be recorded in a simple fourfold table (Table 4.1). The table shows that it is possible to calculate the frequency of different outcomes in two ways. One may do the calculation horizontally and determine, for instance, the rate of true positive results among patients with a positive test, or one may calculate vertically and

Table 4.1 The diagnostic universe.

		Disease		
		Present	Absent	
Diagnostic test	Positive	True positives	False positives	All positives
	Negative	False negatives	True negatives	All negatives
		All with disease	All without disease	

determine, for instance, the rate of true positive results among patients with the disease.

Those rates that are calculated horizontally are called *diagnostic rates*. They are the ones that the diagnostician uses when he sees the test result and wishes to determine the probability that the patient suffers from a particular disease.

Those that are calculated vertically are called *nosographic rates* as they serve to describe the disease in question. The descriptions of different diseases in medical textbooks provide nosographic information, such as information about the frequency of clinical and paraclinical findings among patients with a particular disease.

Table 4.1 therefore permits the calculation of the following eight different rates or probabilities (we assume that the samples are so large that the rates are good approximations to the probabilities). We use the generally accepted notation for conditional probabilities, according to which P(A|B) means the probability of A *if* B.

TP, FP, TN and FN in the following definitions mean true positive, false positive, true negative and false negative. D+ or D− mean presence or absence of disease and T+ and T− mean positive or negative test.

Diagnostic probabilities:

- P(D+|T+) = the diagnostic TP probability, i.e. the probability that a patient has the disease if the test is positive. It is calculated as: number of true positives/total number of positives.

- P(D−|T+) = the diagnostic FP probability, i.e. the probability that a patient does not have the disease if the test is positive. It is calculated as: number of false positives/total number of positives.

- $P(D-|T-)$ = the diagnostic TN probability, i.e. the probability that a patient does not have the disease if the test is negative. It is calculated as: number of true negatives/total number of negatives.

- $P(D+|T-)$ = the diagnostic FN probability, i.e. the probability that a patient has the disease if the test is negative. It is calculated as: number of false negatives/total number of negatives.

Nosographic probabilities:

- $P(T+|D+)$ = the nosographic TP probability, i.e. the probability that a patient with the disease has a positive test result. It is calculated as: number of true positives/total number of patients with the disease.

- $P(T-|D+)$ = the nosographic FN probability, i.e. the probability that a patient with the disease has a negative test result. It is calculated as: number of false negatives/total number of patients with the disease.

- $P(T-|D-)$ = the nosographic TN probability, i.e. the probability that a patient without the disease has a negative test result. It is calculated as: number of true negatives/total number of patients without disease.

- $P(T+|D-)$ = the nosographic FP probability, i.e. the probability that a patient without the disease has a positive test result. It is calculated as: number of false positives/total number of patients without the disease.

The eight probabilities form four complementary pairs, e.g. the diagnostic TP rate $= 1-$ the diagnostic FP probability.

Diagnosis of diseases with an accessible defining criterion

The direct method for assessing the accuracy of test results

This terminology is very useful for the assessment of the accuracy of diagnostic tests if it is possible to establish or exclude the diagnosis with certainty by means of some other method. In other words, it is required that the disease has an accessible defining criterion.

Table 4.2 Ultrasonography for the diagnosis of acute appendicitis. Diagnostic TP and TN rates with 95% confidence intervals are shown.

| | | Final diagnosis Appendicitis | | Total |
		Present	Absent	
Ultrasonography	Positive	45	8	50
	Negative	10	51	61
	Total	52	59	111

$P(D+ \mid T+) = 42/50 = 84.0\%$ (70.9–92.8%)
$P(D- \mid T-) = 51/61 = 83.6\%$ (72.0–91.8%)

Table 4.2 shows the results of a study assessing the accuracy of ultrasonic scanning for the diagnosis of acute appendicitis. One hundred and eleven consecutive patients with a clinical picture suggesting this diagnosis entered the study. They were subjected to sonography, the results of which were labelled positive or negative, and afterwards the true diagnosis was established by inspection during laparotomy. The fourfold table contains the information which is needed for estimating the diagnostic TP probability, $P(D+|T+)$, and the diagnostic TN probability, $P(D-|T-)$. These two probabilities are of paramount importance from a clinical point of view as $P(D+|T+)$ tells us to which extent we may rely on the test when we wish to confirm the diagnosis whereas $P(D-|T-)$ tells us to which extent we may rely on the test when we wish to exclude the diagnosis.

As the number of patients was relatively small, the calculated rates are shown with 95% confidence intervals that indicate where the true rates are likely to be (see Chapter 5).

This was a very simple example, but in practice it is very difficult to avoid methodological problems. Sometimes the diagnostic test provides ambiguous results that cannot simply be classified as positive or negative, and sometimes it proves impossible to establish the final diagnosis. Therefore, a 3×3 table is needed rather than a simple fourfold table. Researchers who have reduced their data to a 2×2 table must therefore always explain which categories they have lumped, and why. We would not like to overlook meningitis, for example, whereas the consequences are less if appendicitis is missed with ultrasound scanning, as the surgeon will proceed with the operation anyhow if the

Table 4.3 Ultrasonography for the diagnosis of acute appendicitis. The actual results of the study are recorded in a 3 × 3 table. Some diagnostic probabilities (with 95% confidence intervals) have been calculated.

		Final diagnosis Appendicitis			
		Present	?	Absent	Total
	Positive	39	4	0	43
Ultrasonography	?	3	1	3	7
	Negative	10	23	28	61
	Total	52	28	31	111

$P(D+\,|\,T+\,) = 39/43 = 90.7\%\ (77.9\text{--}97.4\%)$
$P(D+\,|\,T\,?\,) = 3/7 = 42.9\%\ (9.9\text{--}81.6\%)$
$P(D-\,|\,T-\,) = 28/61 = 45.9\%\ (33.1\text{--}59.2\%)$
$P(D\,?\,|\,T+\,) = 4/43 = 9.8\%\ (2.7\text{--}59.2\%)$

symptoms get worse. If the researchers have not reported any ambiguous results, the reader should suspect that they have omitted these 'inconvenient' data from their paper,[76] although such behaviour, of course, would be a type of scientific misconduct.

The fourfold table in Table 4.2 was based on an actual study, but the recording of the results was simplified in two ways. Firstly, the uncertain results of the ultrasound scanning were recorded as positive and, secondly, those patients who did not undergo a laparotomy were classified as not having appendicitis. Table 4.3 which summarizes the actual results[77] enables us to calculate additional conditional probabilities, such as $P(D+|T?)$, which tells us the probability of appendicitis, if the test result is uncertain.

The method that I have described so far is called the *direct method* for the assessment of diagnostic tests, and the procedure may be summarized as follows:

1. Select a sample of patients with a particular clinical picture;

2. Carry out the diagnostic test and record the results;

3. Establish or exclude the diagnosis by means of another method; and

4. Calculate the diagnostic TP probability and the diagnostic TN probability, i.e. $P(D+|T+)$ and $P(D-|T-)$.

In principle, this is simple, but in practice, it is quite rare that a diagnosis can be established with certainty. It is possible to verify or exclude most cancers through biopsy or operation, whereas it is more uncertain to follow border-line cases for some time without surgery, since some cancers can disappear spontaneously, without treatment.[51]

The indirect method for assessing the accuracy of test results

Another method, which may be called the *indirect or nosographic method*, is also commonly used. Here the procedure is:

1. Select a sample of patients with the disease and a sample of patients without the disease;

2. Carry out the diagnostic test and record the results; and

3. Calculate the nosographic TP probability and the nosographic TN proba-bility, i.e. $P(T+|D+)$ and $P(T-|D-)$.

We may, for instance, imagine that we select 100 patients with the disease in question and 100 without it. Eighty-five of the patients with the disease have a positive test and 95 of the patients without the disease have a negative test. Consequently, the nosographic TP probability is 85% and the nosographic TN probability is 95%. The results are shown in Table 4.4.

These results are only of limited value from a clinical point of view, as the clinician needs to know the diagnostic probabilities. In other words, it is nec-essary to convert the nosographic probabilities into diagnostic probabilities. This can be done if we know the prevalence of the disease, as that informa-tion enables us to calculate the composition of the diagnostic universe. If, for instance, the prevalence of the disease is 10% we may imagine a diagnostic universe comprising 100 patients with the disease (of whom 85% have a posi-tive test) and 900 patients without the disease (of whom 95% have a negative test). This hypothetical example leads to the fourfold table shown as Table 4.5a, which permits a calculation of the relevant diagnostic probabilities. It is seen

Table 4.4 Number of positive and
negative test results (T+ and T−) in
100 patients with the disease (D+) and
100 patients without the disease (D−).

	D+	D−
T+	85	5
T−	15	95
Total	100	100

that the test is only moderately reliable for making the diagnosis as no more than 65.4% of those patients who have a positive test also have the disease, whereas it is much more useful for excluding the diagnosis as 98.3% of the patients with a negative test do not have the disease.

We could also imagine that the prevalence was no more than 1%. This is also a realistic possibility as sometimes we wish to rule out improbable, but serious, diagnoses. In that case we should need 9900 patients to balance the 100 patients with the disease and the result of the calculations are shown in Table 4.5b. Then the test would be useless for establishing the diagnosis as a little less than 15% of patients with a positive test would have the disease, but the reliability of negative test results would be even higher than in the previous example.

Table 4.5c represents the other extreme. Here the prevalence is 80%, which is realistic when we were dealing with a clinical picture that is highly suggestive of one particular disease. Now the test is reliable for confirming the diagnosis as $P(D+|T+)$ is almost 99%, but quite unreliable for excluding the diagnosis, $P(D-|T-)$ being 61.5%.

It is, however, not necessary to construct a fictitious diagnostic universe in order to convert nosographic into diagnostic probabilities. It may also be done by means of Bayes' theorem which in its simplest form looks like this:

$$P(D+|T+) = P(T+|D+)\, \frac{P(D+)}{P(T+)}$$

In this formula $P(D+)$ is the unconditional probability that a patient from this diagnostic universe has the disease, i.e. the disease prevalence, and $P(T+)$ is the unconditional probability that a patient from the universe has a positive

Table 4.5   The diagnostic universe corresponding to the figures in Table 4.4, if the prevalence of the disease is a) 10%, b) 1% and c) 80%. Same notation as in Table 4.4.

a)

	D+	D−	Total
T+	85	45	130
T−	15	855	870
Total	100	900	

$P(D+\,|\,T+) = 85/130 = 65.4\%$
$P(D-\,|\,T-) = 855/870 = 98.3\%$

b)

	D+	D−	Total
T+	85	495	580
T−	15	9405	9420
Total	100	9900	

$P(D+\,|\,T+) = 85/580 = 14.7\%$
$P(D-\,|\,T-) = 9405/9420 = 99.8\%$

c)

	D+	D−	Total
T+	85	1	86
T−	15	24	39
Total	100	25	

$P(D+\,|\,T+) = 85/86 = 98.8\%$
$P(D-\,|\,T-) = 24/39 = 61.5\%$

test. Usually, $P(T+)$ is not known, but then one may use the following more complex formula (where $P(T+)$ is calculated from the available information):

$$P(D+\,|T+) = \frac{P(T+\,|D+)P(D+)}{P(T+\,|D+)P(D+) + P(T+\,|D-)P(D-)}$$

The following calculation of P(D+|T+), which refers to the first of the examples, gives the same result as before (Table 4.5a):

$$P(D+|T+) = \frac{0.85 \times 0.10}{0.85 \times 0.10 + 0.05 \times 0.90} = 0.654$$

P(D−|T−) can be calculated by a similar formula, replacing + by − and vice versa.

The indirect or nosographic method has been discussed in some detail as it illustrates well that the value of the diagnostic probabilities depends on two factors: the nosographic probabilities and the prevalence of the disease. As I shall explain below, Bayesian reasoning is required whenever we wish to use nosographic knowledge (textbook knowledge) for diagnostic purposes.

However, the formal use of the indirect method for the assessment of diagnostic tests is rarely warranted. The procedure suggests that one may determine the nosographic probabilities in one diagnostic universe and then use that information to calculate the diagnostic probabilities in another universe, if one only takes into account the prevalence of the disease. That, however, is not permissible as both the nosographic probabilities and the prevalence differ in different clinical settings. The assessment of a diagnostic test must be confined to one well-defined diagnostic universe. It cannot be taken for granted, for instance, that ultrasound scanning is equally effective for confirming or excluding a diagnosis of pancreatic cancer in patients presenting with abdominal pain, patients presenting with jaundice, and patients presenting with a palpable mass in the abdomen. We must assume that the frequency of positive results among patients with the disease (the nosographic TP rate) differs in these three groups of patients. Similarly, it cannot be assumed that ultrasound scanning is equally effective in general practice as in hospital practice. General practitioners wish to diagnose the early stages of the disease and the small tumours in such patients are more likely to be missed by the ultrasound scan than the larger tumours seen by hospital specialists.

Therefore, it only makes limited sense to discuss in general terms whether or not a particular test is good or bad for diagnosing a particular disease. Usually, one can only tell whether or not the test results are sufficiently accurate either for confirming the diagnosis or for excluding the diagnosis in patients who present a particular clinical picture and who belong to a particular part of the clinical spectrum of the disease.

In other words, we cannot assess a diagnostic test unless we define in advance the diagnostic universe and, when that has been done, it is usually just as easy to select a random sample of patients belonging to that universe and determine directly the diagnostic TP and TN rates. The indirect method is useful if the disease is very rare, as in that case the determination of the diagnostic TP rate, using the direct method, may require a very large sample of patients. It is also useful the first time a new diagnostic test is assessed, since, if the test performs badly under these favourable conditions, there would be little incentive to study its usefulness in realistic clinical situations. As would be expected, comparisons of the two methods have shown that the indirect method produces far more impressive results than the direct method.[78]

There is an increasing interest in the assessment of diagnostic tests, but there is a need for many more studies and for systematic reviews of such studies, as it is currently planned to include in The Cochrane Library (see Chapter 6). The resources of health services are limited and, whenever possible, we ought to assess the accuracy of the new, sometimes very costly, diagnostic techniques before they find their way to the daily routine. It is also to be hoped that the results of the assessments will find their way to the standard textbooks of medicine, which contain little precise information about the value of different tests.

Undoubtedly, many diagnostic tests are much overrated. Gastroenterologists pay much attention to the appearance of the mucosa during gastroduodenoscopy, but a Norwegian population survey of endoscopic and histological findings in people with and without dyspepsia revealed that only 10% in both groups had what was considered a normal mucosa. The endoscopic findings, with the possible exceptions of peptic ulcer disease and endoscopic duodenitis, showed no association of clinical value with dyspepsia.[79]

Terminological confusion

The terminology that has been introduced in this chapter is not generally accepted. The authors of most textbooks on clinical epidemiology and most papers dealing with diagnostic problems write about the specificity and sensitivity of diagnostic tests and the predictive value of positive and negative test results. These terms ('international terminology') are defined as follows:

Specificity = $P(T-|D-)$ (nosographic TN rate)
Sensitivity = $P(T+|D+)$ (nosographic TP rate)
Predictive value of positive test $(PV_{pos}) = P(D+|T+)$ (diagnostic TP rate)
Predictive value of negative test $(PV_{neg}) = P(D-|T-)$ (diagnostic TN rate)

Terminological problems are of course not very interesting *per se* and one may argue that it does not really matter which words we use. In this case, however, the commonly used terms invite misunderstandings.

Only those who have a very good grasp of diagnostic logic will appreciate that in the international terminology the terms specificity and sensitivity have been defined so that they no longer have the same meaning as in ordinary language. If you say, for instance, that a blood test is very specific, you usually mean that you can rely on the positive test results as there will only be few false positive results. In other words, according to the ordinary use of the word, a specific test is a test where the diagnostic TP rate is high, but in the international terminology the specificity is defined as the nosographic TN rate. This is obviously a source of confusion as a high nosographic TN rate need not be associated with a high diagnostic TP rate. In one of the examples above (Table 4.5b) the specificity (using the international definition) was 95%, but the diagnostic TP rate was only about 15%.

Similarly, when we say that a blood test is very sensitive, we usually mean that we can rely on the negative results, i.e. that it rarely fails when the blood contains the substance in question. In other words, according to ordinary usage, a sensitive test is a test where the diagnostic TN rate is high, but in the international terminology it is defined as the nosographic TP rate. That may also lead to misunderstandings. In Table 4.5c the nosographic TP rate was 85%, but the diagnostic TN rate only about 62%.

Frequently it is also suggested that the specificity and sensitivity (i.e. the nosographic probabilities) are stable measures of the reliability of a diagnostic test whereas the diagnostic probabilities are unstable as they depend on the prevalence of the disease. It is this idea that invites the misconception that one may determine the sensitivity and specificity in one clinical setting and then use these results to calculate the diagnostic probabilities for other clinical settings, taking into account the varying prevalence of the disease. As I have explained already this procedure is not acceptable, as nosographic rates, as well as diagnostic rates, depend on the diagnostic universe.

It is also unfortunate that the terms diagnostic and nosographic rates or probabilities have no equivalents in the standard terminology. The false positive rate is a commonly used term, but it is rarely stated how it is calculated, i.e. whether it is the diagnostic or the nosographic FP rate. Many clinicians who hear that the false positive rate is only 5% will believe that then there is only a 5% chance that a patient with a positive test does not have the disease in question but, if the rate is nosographic, that may be a grave misunderstanding. We may again refer to Table 4.5b where the nosographic FP rate was 5% while the diagnostic FP rate was about 85%.

The nosographic rates are of little interest when the clinician seeks the right diagnosis in one of his patients, but they may serve other purposes. Those who plan mass screening for some disease must take into account both the nosographic TP rate and the nosographic FP rate. The former supplies the information how many people with the disease are caught in the net, and the latter how many persons without the disease are also caught. But the interpretation of a test result in the individual case still requires diagnostic thinking. Most people will be impressed when they hear that the sensitivity and specificity of a test used for mass screening are both 98%, but if the prevalence is only 1 per 1000 (which is not unrealistic in a screening project) there is a 95% probability that a patient with a positive test does *not* have the disease.

The international terminology refers to the diagnostic rates as the predictive values of the test, the predictive value of a positive test being the diagnostic TP rate and the predictive value of a negative test being the diagnostic TN rate. That also serves to muddle the thinking. These expressions originated in epidemiology where it is reasonable to talk about the predictive value of different risk factors, but they make no sense in a diagnostic context. Prediction (foretelling) implies reasoning from a causal factor to some possible future effect, but that is not the case when a clinician makes a diagnosis. He analyses the patient's clinical picture and seeks the cause of the observed symptoms and signs; he does not predict anything.

The terminological and conceptual confusion may well explain that few clinicians have a good grasp of diagnostic logic.

Quantitative data

So far we have only considered the assessment of qualitative tests, but many of those diagnostic tests that are used in everyday clinical practice are quantitative. Clinicians, however, do not always quote the exact results when they discuss their patients, but confine themselves to stating that the patient has a low serum potassium, a normal alkaline phosphatase or eosinophilia. They reduce the level of measurement from an interval scale to an ordinal or binary scale, and that, of course, raises the question of how one distinguishes between normal and abnormal (high or low) test results.

Suppose that we wish to assess the value of a quantitative test for the diagnosis of an anatomically defined disease. The reader can probably find an example within his own sphere of interest, e.g. serum alkaline phosphatase for the diagnosis of obstructive jaundice, α-fetoprotein for the diagnosis of hepatocellular carcinoma, or urine catecholamines for the diagnosis of phaeochromocytoma.

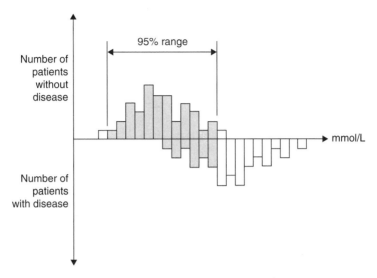

Fig. 4.2   The histogram pointing downwards shows the distribution of the results of a quantitative diagnostic test in patients suffering from a particular disease. The histogram pointing upwards shows the distribution in patients not suffering from the disease.

First, a number of patients suspected of having the disease are collected, then the patients are subjected to the new test and, finally, the true diagnosis is established. Fig. 4.2 shows what the results may look like when the assessment is made of a quantitative blood analysis, the unit of measurement being mmol/L. The histogram pointing upwards shows the distribution of patients who were found not to suffer from the disease in question, and the histogram pointing downwards shows the distribution of patients with the disease. For the sake of simplicity we assume that patients without the disease give the same results as normal people, and in that case the observed 95% range which is shown in the figure is the same as the normal range. It is seen that the new test tends to give higher results in patients with the disease than in patients without the disease, but there is a considerable overlap.

We now wish to draw a line separating normal from high values, assuming that abnormally low values have no clinical significance, and this distinction can be made at different levels. Traditionally, one would prefer to draw the line at the upper limit of the 95% range, and that has been done in Fig. 4.3a where the histogram, for the sake of clarity, has been drawn as a continuous curve. By means of the abscissa axis and the vertical line through the upper limit of the normal range, the patients have been divided into four groups.

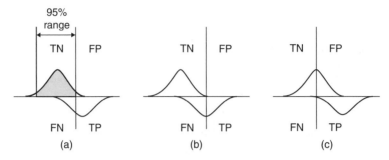

Fig. 4.3 a) Conventional distinction between normal and elevated values. b) Distinction which eliminates false positive results. c) Distinction which eliminates false negative results. For the sake of simplicity, the histograms have been drawn as continuous curves. TN = true negative results, FP = false positive results, FN = false negative results, TP = true positive results.

The upper left quadrant contains those patients who gave a true negative result as the result was negative and the patients did not have the disease. The upper right quadrant contains those patients who gave a false positive result, and they constitute 2.5% of all patients without the disease, as the 95% normal range cuts off the 2.5% highest and the 2.5% lowest values. The lower left quadrant contains the patients with false negative results, and the true positive results are found in the lower right quadrant.

It is also possible to draw the line between normal and elevated values at other levels. In Fig. 4.3b the distinction is made in such a way that all patients without the disease are said to give a normal test result. In that case there will be no false positive results, but in return a large number of patients with the disease present a false negative result.

In Fig. 4.3c we have gone to the other extreme as the line has been drawn in such a way that the test result is said to be elevated in all patients with the disease. Now there are no false negative, but many false positive results.

It is also relevant in this case to distinguish between diagnostic and noso-graphic probabilities. In Fig. 4.3a the number of patients who gave false positive results (the patients in the upper right quadrant) constituted 2.5% of all pa-tients without the disease (all results above the line) and, therefore, 2.5% is the nosographic FP rate. If instead the number of false positive results is related to the total number of positive results (all results to the right of the vertical line), we shall obtain the diagnostic FP rate.

This way of thinking also applies to descriptive qualitative tests. It is, for instance, not possible to distinguish sharply between benign cells and malignant cells in cytological preparations, and by altering the criteria it may be possible to alter the proportion of false positives and false negatives. Stringent criteria give few false positive results and many false negatives, whereas less stringent criteria have the opposite effect.[80]

These examples illustrate that no clear-cut distinction can be made between quantitative and qualitative data. Classification of cells as malignant or benign is, from a formal point of view, a binary scale measurement, but nevertheless there is a gradual transition between the two classes, and it is up to the cytologist to draw the line between them. The potassium concentration of serum is measured on an interval scale, but the physician has to reduce the measurement to a lower level in order to decide if a patient suffers from hyperkaliaemia, has a normal concentration or suffers from hypokaliaemia. The clinician is a decision-maker and before he can take further action he must, as it was once said, choose his operating points on the criterion axis.[4]

Up to now we have only considered the diagnostic importance of single tests, but that is an oversimplification of clinical decision-making. The physician who sees a jaundiced patient will be interested in both the alkaline phosphatase and the aminotransferase. If the aminotransferase level is highly elevated and the alkaline phosphatase is only slightly increased, infectious hepatitis is suspected, and if the opposite is true obstructive jaundice is more likely. Here the physician uses the combination of two quantitative paraclinical findings that have been reduced to an ordinal scale with three classes (normal, slightly elevated, highly elevated), but usually diagnostic reasoning is much more complicated.

Diagnosis of diseases with a concealed defining criterion

So far the value of diagnostic tests has been discussed in probabilistic terms. This approach was illustrated by a number of numerical examples, but they were all based on the assumption that the truth of the diagnosis could be established by independent means. This assumption, however, is rarely fulfilled in practice, and in actual fact we have only been dealing with ideal cases. If the disease has a concealed defining criterion, the true diagnosis may never be revealed.

Myocardial and pulmonary infarction are typical examples of diseases with a concealed defining criterion. A textbook author once wrote that the discovery of increased concentrations of some enzymes in patients with myocardial infarction 'ushered in a new era of diagnostic accuracy' and the same could have been said about the introduction of pulmonary scintigraphy for the diagnosis of infarctions in the lungs. On reflection it will be found that such statements are not quite as simple as they sound. Imagine, for instance, that we wanted to assess the diagnostic accuracy of an elevated MB (myocardial band) isoenzyme of creatine phosphokinase for diagnosing myocardial infarction. According to the direct method, the procedure would be as follows: first, some patients are selected who are suspected of having a myocardial infarction, for instance patients who developed sudden praecordial pain. Next, the serum content of the enzyme is determined, and a distinction is made between a normal and an elevated concentration. Then, however, we run into difficulties, as fortunately most of the patients survive, and in all those cases we shall not know with absolute certainty whether or not the patient had an infarction, and therefore we shall never learn whether the test result was true or false. It is impossible to calculate the diagnostic TP and TN rates, if the defining criterion remains concealed, and instead it is necessary to substantiate the accuracy of the test results by indirect means. This can be done in a number of different ways.

Firstly, we may rely on our knowledge of anatomy and physiology and of the pathogenesis of the disease. We know that the heart muscle is damaged by the blocked blood flow and we understand that this may have the effect that enzymes normally found in the heart leak into the blood. We also know that the MB-isoenzyme is found only in the heart whereas other isoenzymes of creatine phosphokinase are also present in skeletal muscle. Therefore, it is reasonable to expect that the diagnostic TP rate will be higher if we only determine the MB-isoenzyme. However, we must ascertain that the laboratory techniques that are used for isolating the isoenzyme are sufficiently specific.

Similarly, we may deduce from our theoretical knowledge that combined pulmonary perfusion and ventilation scintigraphy is a useful test. I shall not go into details, but just sketch the flow of the reasoning. The technetium^{99m}-labelled particles that are infused are caught in the pulmonary capillary bed, and normally the scintigram exhibits a homogeneous distribution of radioactivity in the lungs. In pulmonary infarction, however, the blood flow to some section of the lung will be blocked, and a 'defect' with absent radioactivity will be seen. Therefore, it is assumed that the diagnostic TN probability is high, but it is not assumed that the diagnostic TP probability is also high, as other lung diseases may also cause local disturbances of the blood flow. To solve this problem a ventilation test is carried out where the patient inhales a radioactive gas. Pulmonary embolism does not reduce the ventilation of the affected zone and therefore the ventilation scintigram will be normal. Consequently, the two tests are interpreted together and it is assumed that the diagnostic TP probability is high, if the perfusion scan is positive and the ventilation scan negative.

It is this kind of reasoning that has led to the introduction of these and many other tests, and although the flow of the arguments may seem very logical, they only provide sophisticated circumstantial evidence. In the case of pulmonary scintigraphy, we cannot be sure that small infarctions are always detected or that the ventilation scan is always normal in other diseases, and we know that the inter-observer variation may be considerable (see Chapter 2). Therefore, there can be little doubt that in clinical practice we encounter both false positive and false negative results, but since the defining criterion in most cases remains concealed, we do not know how often this happens.

If the patient dies and an autopsy is performed, the defining criterion becomes accessible, and usually the diagnosis that was made when the patient was alive is confirmed. Then it is tempting to conclude that the results of the test are also accurate in those patients who survive, but that is of course not certain. Patients may die from a myocardial or a pulmonary infarction, but perhaps the fatality rate of those conditions that mimic these diseases clinically is low, and in that case the false positive results will not be detected at the autopsy table.

Extrapolation from patients who die to patients who survive was first introduced by the French pathologists at the beginning of the nineteenth century, and it was also used by With in his treatise on gastric ulcer in 1881 (p. 45). He observed that those young women who were admitted because of an acute abdominal crisis, and died, had a gastric ulcer, and since many of them presented a history of epigastric pain he assumed that other young women with epigastric pain also had a gastric ulcer. He was probably right, but it cannot be proved.

This does not imply, of course, that observations made at the autopsy table are of little interest. On the contrary, they are very important, as they serve to confront the clinician with his diagnostic mistakes. Until a few decades ago autopsies were done almost routinely in many European countries. Every time a patient died the clinicians who had treated the patient visited the pathology department and inspected the organs. Now, the autopsy rate has dropped drastically, which must mean that some diagnostic errors never come to light. This may enhance clinicians' tendency to overestimate the accuracy of the tests that they use.

Sometimes when it is not possible to establish the diagnosis with certainty, it is decided to circumvent the problems by choosing a *gold standard*. In other words, the results of the new test are compared with the results of some other test, which is considered reliable, but may have the disadvantage that it is more expensive or unpleasant for the patients. There are, for instance, a number of studies where the results of pulmonary scintigraphy are compared with the results of pulmonary angiography. This is not an unreasonable idea, but it is far from certain that the reliability of angiography is perfect, as regards reproducibility and accuracy. If the result of one method is positive and that of the other negative, it is not certain which is correct and which is wrong.

The course of the disease and the combined results of other tests may also provide a gold standard. This procedure was used in the case of the MB-isoenzyme. This test is considered useful for establishing or excluding the diagnosis of a myocardial infarction at a very early stage, and its reliability for that purpose could be assessed by relating the results to the final diagnosis after prolonged observation of the symptoms, the ECG changes and the changes of the levels of other enzymes.[81]

In practice, the diagnosis of diseases with a concealed defining criterion also involves simple pattern recognition. Clinicians may regard the diseases as clinical syndromes, which means that they take into account all the clinical data, including symptoms, signs and paraclinical findings, and make the diagnosis if the total clinical picture is sufficiently typical. If, however, diagnosis is viewed from this angle, we face other, equally difficult, problems.

Syndrome diagnosis

Many years ago, at a clinical conference, a chemical pathologist proposed a new serological test for the diagnosis of infectious mononucleosis. He said that Paul Bunnel's test, which was the only one used at that time, was positive only in 70% of cases, whereas the new test was positive in 90% of cases. A critical clinician pondered over this information and replied rather unkindly: 'If it is possible to calculate these percentages, then there must be a third method by which the diagnosis can be made with 100% certainty. We should like to hear more about this third method and discuss its introduction.' There was, of course, no such method, as infectious mononucleosis at that time (before the importance of Epstein–Barr virus was recognized) must be regarded as an undefined, or at most arbitrarily defined, clinical syndrome, and the percentages mentioned did not prove the superiority of the new test.

One might also have raised another equally justified objection. The quoted percentages represent nosographic TP rates, and as explained above, it is necessary to determine also the nosographic TN rate, and especially the relevant diagnostic rates.

A paper was published recommending a new method of diagnosing hyperthyroidism[82] in much the same manner. The author had collected a group of patients in whom the diagnosis had been made using all available diagnostic tests, including the new one. He then calculated which test was positive in the greatest number of cases, and *mirabile dictu* the new test won the competition. The only conclusion that can be drawn from such a study is that the author attached more importance to the results of the new test than to the results of the others, when he made the diagnosis. It is important that the consumer of medical literature is not deceived when medical writers use circular arguments.

Doctors still make similar mistakes as they have little training in analysing such logical problems of syndrome diagnosis (including metabolically defined diseases which are treated like clinical syndromes), but it is much easier to criticize than to be constructive. Where clinical syndromes are concerned it is difficult to lay down clear-cut principles for the assessment of new diagnostic methods.

One may say that syndrome diagnosis is simply a matter of pattern recognition. If we assume that all common syndromes are well defined, the diagnosis of a syndrome simply consists of the demonstration of those clinical data that must be present according to the syndrome definition. According to this point of view, the diagnostic tests only serve to fill in the patient's clinical picture, and it has little meaning to discuss the probability of the diagnosis. If, for instance, a patient fulfils the criteria of rheumatoid arthritis mentioned on p. 50, then he has got the disease, and if he does not fulfil the criteria he has not got the disease. It is a case of all or nothing and not a question of probabilities.

This presentation, however, oversimplifies matters, because in everyday clinical medicine, syndrome diagnosis undoubtedly includes a probabilistic element.

When the clinician has recorded his patient's iatrotropic symptoms and the usual routine data, he will consider which diagnosis is the most probable, and if this diagnosis is a clinical syndrome, he will institute those investigations that are necessary to fill in the clinical picture. If the patient does not fulfil the criteria for that syndrome, he will then institute those investigations that are needed to make or exclude the second most probable disease, and so on.

Most syndromes, however, are not well defined, and even if they were, there would still be patients who would only fulfil some of the criteria for that particular syndrome. When that is the case the clinician must decide if he still wants to make the diagnosis, i.e. if he still wants to treat the patient as if all the criteria were fulfilled. It is, for instance, not unusual at a rheumatological department that a patient is thought to have a so-called connective tissue disease, although the serological reactions and the skin and muscle biopsies have not provided results which fulfil all the accepted diagnostic criteria for any syndrome belonging to that group of diseases. In such a case it may still be reasonable to start treatment with corticosteroids, because it is considered likely that the patient has a connective tissue disease after all, which really means that probably the patient will respond to treatment in the same way as those patients who fulfil all the criteria.

It is important to understand how syndromes are first described, and how they change. Rheumatoid arthritis may again serve as an example as we still do not know enough about the disease mechanisms to be able to suggest a pathogenetic or an aetiological definition.

This syndrome was originally introduced because clinicians had observed patients with clinical pictures which resembled each other to such an extent that it was considered justified to say that they had the same disease. Such clinical pictures characterized by symptoms and clinical signs formed the original nucleus of the syndrome, and the patients in question may be regarded as 'typical' cases of rheumatoid arthritis. They are represented by the circular area A in Fig. 4.4a. In addition, 'atypical' cases were observed, i.e. patients whose clinical pictures to a varying extent differed from the 'typical' pictures. If the difference was small, the patients were still said to have rheumatoid arthritis (the annular area B in Fig. 4.4a), and if the difference was larger this diagnosis was not made (area C in Fig. 4.4a). Thus, the final result is that the grey area of the figure comprises patients who were given the diagnosis of rheumatoid arthritis. The boundary between these categories of patients was of course not sharp, but the example serves to illustrate the principles of syndrome diagnosis on purely clinical criteria.

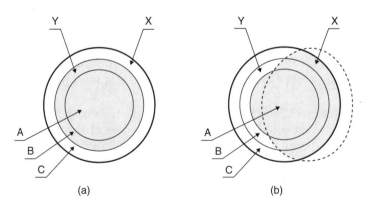

Fig. 4.4 Diagnosis of rheumatoid arthritis before (a) and after (b) the introduction of a new serological diagnostic test. See text for further explanation. X and Y represent two patients whose diagnosis was affected by the introduction of the new test.

In the 1930s it was discovered that serum from patients with rheumatoid arthritis frequently contained agglutinins against haemolytic streptococci, and the agglutination reaction became accepted as a diagnostic test. The resulting influence on the diagnosis of the syndrome is shown in Fig. 4.4b, in which the oval figure represents all patients with a positive test.

Patients with typical clinical pictures (area A) still received the diagnosis of rheumatoid arthritis, since it may be presumed that a negative result of the new test would not make the clinician reject the diagnosis when the clinical evidence was strong. In patients with atypical pictures (areas B and C), however, the test must have influenced the diagnosis, because it was in these cases that the clinician needed the additional paraclinical evidence. If he relied on the test, which he probably did as he used it, we may presume that he made a diagnosis of rheumatoid arthritis if the test was positive and that he did not make the diagnosis if it was negative. The situation is illustrated by Fig. 4.4b, where the grey area shows which patients were labelled as having rheumatoid arthritis after the introduction of the test. The net result was that the use of the diagnostic term had changed.

This test is now obsolete, but others have replaced it as diagnostic aids, and one may assume that each time the syndrome diagnosis was affected. This situation was foreseen by the American Rheumatism Association. When they first established a set of criteria they commented that it must be revised from time to time so that the definition does not become outdated.[83] Later, it was discovered that many clustered cases of arthritis among young people were caused by infection with a bacterium, *Borrelia burgdorferi*, and these cases were therefore separated as a new disease entity.

This example illustrates the fundamental difference between the use of diagnostic tests in clinical syndromes and in, for instance, anatomically defined diseases with an accessible defining criterion. We cannot assess the tests that we use for the diagnosis of clinical syndromes by quoting the diagnostic TP and TN rates as we ourselves determine the accuracy of the results. If we usually make the diagnosis when the test is positive and usually exclude the diagnosis when the test is negative, we shall, of course, find that the diagnostic rates are high. Many tests used in the daily routine have probably been introduced in this dubious manner, and once they have been accepted we soon feel that we cannot do without them.

The introduction of new tests may be prompted by our more or less well-founded hypotheses about the aetiology and pathogenesis of the disease, but we must always ask ourselves if they are really necessary. Unnecessary changes of the diagnostic criteria have the unfortunate consequence that past clinical experience may become outdated. If the current diagnostic criteria no longer correspond to those entry criteria that were used in the randomized trials (see Chapter 6), the results of these trials may become less useful.

Three patients

The analysis of the diagnostic decision on the preceding pages may be summarized by means of three clinical cases where two skilled clinicians disagree about the diagnosis.

The first patient is admitted with an acute abdomen. One clinician believes that the patient has an acute appendicitis, whereas his colleague does not think that this is the case. Here, one clinician is right and the other is wrong, and if they agree on doing a laparotomy and open the patient's abdomen we shall soon find out who is right and who is wrong. The defining criterion becomes accessible at the operation.

The second patient suddenly developed praecordial pain. All the necessary investigations are done, including ECGs and enzyme tests, but the two clinicians read the evidence differently. One believes that the patient has a myocardial infarction and the other does not think so. In this case, too, one clinician must be right and the other wrong, but if the patient gets well and is discharged from hospital some days later we shall never learn the truth. The defining criterion remains concealed.

The third patient has a complex clinical picture with muscular weakness and a skin eruption. The necessary investigations are done, including skin and muscle biopsies. One clinician believes that it is a case of dermatomyositis, while the other denies this. In this case it makes little sense to say that one is right and the other wrong, as dermatomyositis is a clinical syndrome for which no generally accepted set of diagnostic criteria exists. We must simply conclude that these two rheumatologists define the syndrome differently. They may, however, decide to see the patient at regular intervals, and if the patient later develops a clinical picture which is so typical that it is recognized by everybody, we may conclude in retrospect which rheumatologist made the right diagnosis.

These three patients summarize the fundamental logical problems that we face whenever we try to assess the accuracy of the diagnostic methods that we use. Methodological standards for evaluation of diagnostic tests have been developed,[84] but surveys have revealed that only a small minority of papers dealing with the assessment of diagnostic methods are methodologically acceptable.[85,86] Many studies are seriously biased, exhibit circular logic, misinterpret the calculated probabilities or ignore patients with uncertain test results. Typically, the indirect method is used and only the nosographic probabilities (sensitivity and specificity) are quoted, even in diseases, such as temporal arteritis[87] where information about the diagnostic FN probability is essential due to the dire consequence, loss of vision, of missing the diagnosis.

Some of the problems reflect the nature of the disease classification, but in those cases where it is impossible to establish the truth of the test results, we should remember that the diagnosis is not an end in itself. The diagnostic decision is only, as it was once said, a mental resting place on the way to treatment. If we accept this way of thinking, the truth of the diagnosis becomes less important, and we may instead try to assess whether the introduction of the new test improves the treatment results. Years ago, before the routine use of pulmonary scintigraphy for the diagnosis of pulmonary infarction, one might have done a large randomized clinical trial (see Chapter 6) of patients with clinical pictures suggesting this diagnosis. Then treatment in one group might be instituted on the basis of the clinical findings and in the other on the basis of the scintigrams and the clinical findings. If the patients in the latter group fared better, one would have proved that the introduction of this diagnostic procedure was beneficial. Otherwise, it would have been shown to be superfluous. There can be no doubt that the ideal way of assessing the value of a diagnostic test is to subject it to a randomized clinical trial, but this is rarely done.

Diagnosis in practice

Frequential and subjective probabilities

In this chapter the words probabilistic and probability have been used repeatedly. In the numerical example in Table 4.5a the diagnostic TP probability was 65.4% and the diagnostic TN probability was 98.3%. Later, it was stated that there might be a 95% probability that an individual taking part in a screening project does not have the disease, in spite of the fact that the test result is positive, and it was mentioned in connection with syndrome diagnosis that the clinician facing an individual patient must always consider the probability of different diagnostic options.

These statements may seem quite straightforward, but in fact they represent two very different probability concepts as the diagnostic probabilities in the first two statements refer to groups of patients, whereas the probabilities in last two statements refer to individual patients.[7] I shall briefly consider this theoretical question as it serves to clarify a fundamental problem in evidence-based medicine. It helps to explain what it means to make decisions about the individual patient on the basis of experience that has been gained by studying groups of patients.

When we talk about diagnostic or nosographic probabilities we use the traditional frequential or statistical probability concept as the probability represents the 'true' frequency in the population. If we say, for instance, that the diagnostic TP probability is 80%, we mean that the frequency of patients with the disease is 80% in a population of people with a positive test. In practice, we determine the diagnostic TP rate (or frequency) in a limited sample of patients, but for the sake of simplicity we take it for granted in this discussion that the sample is so large that we can ignore the difference between the observed and the true rate.

If, however, we say that there is an 80% probability that a particular patient has the disease, we must mean something else. It cannot be a frequency as it makes no sense to say that the frequency of the disease in one patient is 80%. The patient either has or does not have the disease. Here we use the subjective probability concept, where the probability expresses our degree of confidence in the presence or absence of a particular phenomenon. When we say that there is an 80% probability that a patient suffers from a particular disease, we mean that we are 80% confident that this is the case.

Our justification for that degree of confidence may well be that we have read a paper in a medical journal which reported that the diagnostic TP rate among patients presenting similar clinical pictures was 80%, and in that case the argument goes as follows: The subjective probability of (our confidence in) the diagnosis in this patient is 80% as the frequential probability of the diagnosis among similar patients with a positive test is 80%.

This analysis may seem pedantic, but it is important, as it leaves room for the individualization of clinical reasoning. Perhaps the clinician possesses additional information about the patient. There may have been other cases of the disease in the family, and if it is known to be hereditary he might conclude that in this particular case his confidence in the diagnosis is not 80%, but 95%.

The subjective probability concept is of particular interest when we are dealing with diseases with a concealed defining criterion. Imagine a physician who sees a patient with symptoms suggesting pulmonary embolism whose pulmonary scintigraphy shows the typical 'mismatch' between the perfusion and ventilation scans. He will say that there is almost a 100% probability that this patient has a pulmonary infarction, but this time the subjective probability is not based on an observed frequency, as in most cases the diagnosis remains concealed. His confidence in the diagnosis is based on knowledge of the pathogenesis of the disease and the theoretical rationale of the two forms of scintigraphy.

Diagnostic strategy

I should have liked to explain in detail how clinicians think when they examine their patients and seek the right diagnosis, but unfortunately nobody has ever been able to do so. Diagnostic reasoning is extremely complex, and I shall only be able to discuss this topic in general terms.

The clinician starts thinking about the diagnosis as soon as he has seen the patient and the patient has revealed his complaints (the iatrotropic symptoms). In some cases he will immediately make a diagnosis by simple pattern recognition (e.g. the zoster case mentioned at the beginning of this chapter), but usually the diagnostic process is hypothetico-deductive. We may teach medical students to take a full history and to do a complete physical examination, but the experienced clinician will soon generate diagnostic hypotheses that he then seeks to confirm or exclude by specific questions, by the physical examination and by paraclinical tests.

In this respect diagnostic thinking resembles scientific thinking, as scientists engaged in innovative research will also generate hypotheses that they then subject to critical experiments. This analogy is interesting from the point of view that the mental process involved in the generation of scientific hypotheses is quite unknown and the same can be said about the generation of diagnostic hypotheses. The ability to make fruitful conjectures varies among scientists, and similar variation among doctors may help to explain that some are better diagnosticians than others. Obviously, theoretical knowledge and experience are also important as the clinician can only think of those diseases with which he is acquainted.

Diagnostic reasoning always includes probabilistic considerations. The initial diagnostic hypotheses, i.e. the tentative diagnoses, are all, to a varying extent, probable, and, gradually, the clinician must shorten the list of diagnostic possibilities. In complicated cases simple tests that provide reliable negative results may be used to eliminate some of the tentative diagnoses, and afterwards, when only few possibilities remain, more sophisticated tests that provide reliable positive results may be used to establish the final diagnosis.

The probabilistic considerations will rarely be exact, but there can be no doubt that the good diagnostician, even if he has never heard the expression, is an expert in Bayesian thinking. To explain that, we shall once again look at Bayes' formula in its simple form. $T+$ in this context may represent not only a positive test result, but also a particular clinical picture or a particular symptom or sign:

$$P(D+ | T+) = P(T+ | D+) \frac{P(D+)}{P(T+)}$$

The formula shows that in order to determine the probability of a particular diagnosis the clinician must be able to assess: a) the probability of the clinical picture in question among patients with that disease, i.e. the nosographic TP probability or $P(T+|D+)$; b) the probability that a patient in his practice has the disease (*the practice prevalence*), i.e. $P(D+)$; and c) the probability that one of his patients presents that particular clinical picture, i.e. $P(T+)$.

The probability that an individual patient suffers from a particular disease, $P(D+|T+)$, is a subjective probability, but it is derived from the assessment of three frequential probabilities. Once again we are faced with the typical situation that a clinician uses his empirical knowledge about groups of patients to judge what is the matter with the individual patient.

The first of the three probabilities represents the clinician's nosographic knowledge, which he may have obtained by reading about the clinical presentation of the disease in the appropriate chapter of a medical textbook. When it is mentioned that a particular symptom, sign or clinical picture is very common, common or rare, those statements may be regarded as inexact nosographic TP probabilities. The two other probabilities are rarely recorded anywhere and the clinician must rely on his uncontrolled experience.

As mentioned already the patients described in the textbooks may not correspond to those seen by the clinician, but nevertheless Bayesian thinking is required whenever textbook knowledge is used for diagnosing individual patients, and clinicians must be aware of the implications of this fact. It is, for instance, a common experience that newly fledged general practitioners tend to believe that their patients suffer from all sorts of rare diseases. They have had most of their training as junior hospital doctors and if one of them has recently been employed at a gastroenterological hospital department he may well suspect that Crohn's disease is the most probable diagnosis in a patient with chronic diarrhoea. He is still programmed with the relatively high $P(D+)$ for that disease at the hospital and therefore he overestimates $P(D+|T+)$. Similar problems arise when a doctor trained in Europe moves, for instance, to Tanzania. He may have learnt his textbook on tropical diseases by heart, but he will not be a good diagnostician until he has also learnt to assess correctly the frequency of different diseases and the frequency of different clinical pictures in that part of the world.

This presentation might give the impression that the clinician's degree of confidence in a particular diagnosis, i.e. the subjective probability of the diagnosis, is only based on frequential considerations, but I have mentioned already that this is not the case. The diagnostic strategy also includes deductive reasoning from theoretical knowledge. At the beginning of this chapter I mentioned the jaundiced patient where the consultant deduced from his knowledge about the excretion of bilirubin what might be wrong with the patient. In that case the list of tentative diagnoses was the result of deductive thinking. We may assume that the consultant proceeded by ordering the appropriate blood tests and an ultrasound scan of the liver, and then by a combination of deductive and probabilistic reasoning reached the final diagnosis.

The choice of diagnostic strategy is further complicated by the fact that the clinician must take into account, not only the probability that the patient suffers from different diseases, but also the consequences for the patient of making or not making a diagnosis. In some cases the consequences of missing a diagnosis are so grave that it must be excluded even in those cases where it is highly improbable. It may be considered necessary to do a lumbar puncture in a febrile patient to exclude an unlikely diagnosis of meningitis or to examine the colon of a patient with a fairly typical irritable bowel syndrome in order to exclude that the symptoms are caused by a colonic cancer.

In other cases the probability of a disease may be rather high, but it may still not be justified to pursue that diagnosis. This would be the case if a chest X-ray reveals a shadow in the lung that might well be caused by a cancer, if the patient's clinical condition prohibits further action. There seems to be a tendency in contemporary practice to subject old patients to too many diagnostic investigations of no consequence. Sometimes truth is stronger than fiction. In USA about half of those women who were at least 80 years of age had attended screening for breast cancer with mammography within the last two years,[88] even though there can be no doubt that the harms of screening by far exceed the benefits in this age group.[53]

The clinician must also take into account other consequences of his decisions. Some diagnostic procedures are unpleasant for the patient and may even lead to complications, and others are expensive.

Diagnostic strategy is often a balancing act. The clinician must not overlook diseases in need of treatment and he must not make a diagnosis when it is not warranted. Meador once reported a particularly crude example of overdiagnosis[89,90] or, to use his own expression, the tendency to make a diagnosis of 'nondisease' which is then used to justify a therapeutic decision. In the 1930s, 1000 school children in New York were seen sequentially by four different groups of doctors who were unaware of the fact that the children had been seen or would be seen by other doctors. The first group of doctors found that 611 of the 1000 children had undergone tonsillectomy or were in need of that operation. The second group of doctors saw the remaining 389 children and judged that 174 of them were in need of tonsillectomy, and then the residual 215 children were seen by the third group of doctors who advised tonsillectomy on an additional 99. The last 116 children were seen by the fourth group who suggested tonsillectomy in 65. Now only 51 of the 1000 children were left.

There are other historical examples of nondisease, such as the diagnosis of gastroptosis, an elongated colon or chronic appendicitis, and possibly the recent diagnosis 'chronic fatigue syndrome' belongs to the same category. This is a controversial issue, and I do not deny that some virus infections are followed by a prolonged period of fatigue, but in many cases the justification of this diagnostic label seems doubtful. Patients with psychosocial problems often receive unwarranted somatic diagnoses although, usually, they are less fanciful than this new syndrome.

The inherent complexity of diagnostic reasoning explains that the diagnostic process cannot be reduced to a simple algorithm and it was only to be expected that, so far, computer diagnosis has not been much of a success. It also explains that diagnostic skills cannot be learnt from textbooks alone, but also require bedside teaching.

5

Uncontrolled Experience

Errare humanum est sed in errore perseverare turpe
(To err is human but to repeat the error is shameful)

Old saying

Treatment may take many forms, from advice about change of lifestyle to drug therapy and surgery, and the objects of therapeutic decisions are equally varied. We use such terms as symptomatic, causal, curative, palliative and prophylactic treatment, and clinicians must always bear in mind what effect they wish to obtain by a given intervention. In bronchial asthma, for instance, they may treat patients with bronchodilating agents or corticosteroids either to stop the acute attack or to prevent new attacks, and they may treat cancer patients with surgery either to cure or to palliate.

Clinicians must also consider why they expect a treatment to have the desired effect, and here there are three possibilities:

1. Deduction from theory. Theoretical knowledge of disease mechanisms and the mechanism of action of the treatment in question makes the clinician believe that the treatment is effective.

2. Uncontrolled experience. The clinician herself and other clinicians are convinced, by their everyday experience, that the treatment is effective.

3. Controlled experience. Well-controlled clinical research, preferably in the form of randomized clinical trials, has provided convincing evidence that the treatment is effective.

We are, of course, on very firm ground if we know how the treatment works, if there is a consensus of opinion that it does work, and if randomized clinical trials have given the expected results, but unfortunately this ideal requirement is rarely fulfilled. Therefore, it is necessary to discuss separately the three possible reasons for expecting a therapeutic response, and in this connection we should not forget the lesson of medical history.

Uncontrolled experience in a pre-scientific era

There are many examples that the uncontrolled experience of both medical doctors and lay people has made important contributions to clinical medicine, and I shall mention a few of these.

The story of scurvy is a good example of the inertia of medical progress in former days.[91] The toll of this disease was extremely heavy when the Europeans began to explore the world across the oceans; on some of the longest sea voyages the majority of the seamen died. The Spaniards and the Dutch had noted the effect of lemons as early as the sixteenth century and so did Richard Hawkins and James Lancaster about 1600, but for a long time this uncontrolled experience did not gain general recognition. In 1747 James Lind did an experiment where 12 patients with scurvy received different treatments; only two of these, who were given lemons and oranges, improved. Lind himself was not convinced, but the same year John Huxham reported that, in contrast to ordinary seamen, officers who carried wine, cider, lemons and fresh provisions did not get scurvy. He also described how the disease was cured when the seamen reached harbour and got 'proper food and herbage'.[62] Finally, in 1795 the Admiralty ordered the issue of lemon juice in the Royal Navy.

Popular medicine has also provided effective treatments. In the eighteenth century an old woman in Shropshire observed that a drug containing more than 20 different herbs had a beneficial effect on dropsy,[92] and the general practitioner, William Withering, found that the active component was foxglove (*Digitalis purpurea*). In 1785 he described the effect in a number of cases, including this one: 'A man about fifty years of age ... complained to me of an asthma... His breath was very short, his countenance was sunken, his belly large; and upon examination a fluctuation in it was very perceptible. His urine for some time past had been small in quantity. I directed a decoction of Fo. Digital. recent. which made him very sick, the sickness occurring at intervals for several days, during which time he made a large quantity of water. His breath gradually drew easier, his belly subsided, and in about ten days he begun to eat with a keen appetite'.[62]

The introduction of vaccination against smallpox has an important place in the history of prophylaxis. It was prompted by the experience that people who had had cowpox were spared during smallpox epidemics. Jenner, who in 1798 had practised vaccination for some years, applied for permission to present his results to the Royal Society in London. This request was refused, because 'he ought not to risk his reputation by presenting to the learned body anything which appeared so much at variance with established knowledge and withal so incredible'.[93] However, as it often happens in the history of medicine, 'the established knowledge' was disproved, and this new preventive treatment soon received widespread acceptance.

These examples illustrate that the uncontrolled experience of doctors and laymen have made important contributions to clinical practice, and they also inspired theoretical research. Vaccination against smallpox became the forerunner of immunization against many infectious diseases, and the treatment of scurvy ultimately led to the discovery of vitamins. We usually talk of basic research in the laboratory and applied research at the bedside, but in these cases the situation was reversed.

These examples may well give the impression that the history of medicine is a success story, but we must not forget the seamy side of clinical practice in former days. It was realized even at the time of Hippocrates that clinical experience may be fallacious (*experientia fallax est*), and there seems to be no limit to the number of absurd and often harmful treatments that doctors have used in the course of time.

The Frenchman Amboise Paré, who for a time was a military surgeon, followed the usual routine of treating gunshot wounds by cauterization with boiling oil. However, during a campaign in Italy in 1536, he ran out of oil and instead he had to apply some indifferent concoction. He lay sleepless all night fearing the fate of the unfortunate soldiers who had been treated so unconventionally, and he was much surprised the next morning when he found these soldiers 'free from vehemencie of paine to have had good rest', whereas those soldiers who had been treated correctly were feverish and tormented with pain. Until then numerous soldiers had been exposed to the barbarity of cauterization with a hot iron or with boiling oil. One of the less edifying of Hippocrates' aphorisms runs as follows: 'What medicine does not cure is cured by the knife, what the knife does not cure, is cured by the iron, and what the iron does not cure must be considered incurable'.[94,95]

Enemata were already popular in ancient Egypt, and according to Pliny the enema originated from the observation that the ibis used its curved beak to give itself rectal infusions of Nile water.[94] Since then a variety of rectal infusions have been used in a variety of diseases. In the seventeenth century, rectal infusion of wine was used against consumption, urine enemata were used against dropsy, and holy water enemata were used to exorcize devils from possessed nuns. In the eighteenth century tobacco-smoke clysters were recommended for the resuscitation of drowned persons.

Blood-letting and leeching is a chapter in itself. From classical antiquity to the nineteenth century, blood-letting performed in a variety of ways was a standard treatment of almost any disease. Broussais (1772–1838), who was a highly esteemed professor of pathology in Paris, has been called the most sanguinary physician in history.[94] During the cholera epidemic in 1832 he advocated that the patients were treated with a strict diet and blood-letting by phlebotomy and leeching. A strict diet meant that the patients were not allowed to eat or drink. It has been calculated that 85 000 litres of blood were let at Parisian hospitals in the year 1800;[8] in 1824 France imported 33 million leeches[92] and the British Isles bought 5 million.[94] Leeches have been used far into the twentieth century.

The perusal of any old textbook of medicine reveals page after page of meaningless and harmful treatments. Of course, we cannot know with certainty whether some of the herbs had pharmacological effects which are unknown to us, but by and large we must presume that medical treatment with few exceptions, such as the use of opiates, was quite useless until the end of the nineteenth century. One cannot imagine, for example, that any beneficial effect was obtained by the treatment of a mad dog's bite with angelica root,[21] diabetes or piss-pot disease with burnt hedgehog (eighteenth-century England) or gastric ulcer with cantharides (nineteenth-century Denmark).[68]

The numerical method

At the beginning of the nineteenth century all treatment was still based on speculative theories about the causes of disease and uncontrolled experience, but scientific thinking slowly gained ground. The foundation of modern statistics had been laid, and in the 1830s the first attempts were made to apply statistical methods to clinical medicine. This happened in Paris, and Gavaret's book from 1840 about the principles for the use of statistics in medicine[96] is still very exciting reading. He introduced the concept of confidence intervals, and in 10 tenets he warned clinicians against drawing conclusions from therapeutic experience based on small numbers of patients. The sixth tenet states: 'In order to prefer one therapeutic method to another, the results must not only be better, but the difference must exceed a certain limit which depends on the number of the collected cases'. This book, which includes tables for the calculation of confidence intervals, is more than a hundred years ahead of its time. Gavaret's novel ideas spread to other countries in Europe, and in Denmark, for instance, they had some impact. A young Danish doctor, C.E. Fenger, who later became Minister of Finance, had heard Gavaret's lectures in Paris, and on his return in 1839 he wrote two papers on *the numerical method* in the newly started Danish Medical Journal.[97] He was depressed by the state of contemporary clinical medicine and believed that greater stringency could only be achieved by the introduction of statistical methods. He used pneumonia as an example, and made a critical analysis of diagnosis, prognosis and treatment in numerical terms. He calculated conditional probabilities and stressed that prognostic studies must be related to the clinical pattern. However, the idea that progress in clinical medicine is dependent on observations made with 'order and care on a sufficient number of exactly recorded cases' was too revolutionary for some contemporary colleagues. A regimental surgeon rushed into print with a letter to the editor. The numerical method, he wrote, contains something good and something new. 'What a shame that the good is not new and that the new is not good'. He asserted that the numerical method lets quantity outweigh quality; it ignores the individuality of patients and underrates the experience of skilled clinicians. Similar arguments are still heard nowadays from those who are opposed to evidence-based medicine.

That debate in France and abroad started a development that in the long run proved to be self-effacing. P.C.A. Louis had, for a number of years, studied the prognosis of patients with acute infectious diseases who were bled either earlier or later during the course of their disease. He found that the prognosis did not depend on the time of the phlebotomy and concluded in his book, published in 1835, that blood-letting had only small influence on the course of pneumonia, erysipelas and diphtheria.[98] He did not perform randomized trials, but his observations were felt to be convincing and created great uneasiness in the medical world. The dogma that patients with acute infections had to be bled as quickly as possible had been universally accepted, and now Louis cast doubt on this mainstay of therapy.

One might have expected that the adherents of the numerical school would have begun to test critically all the treatments they used, but that did not happen. Instead, they simply lost faith in their therapeutic remedies, and clinical medicine entered a period that has aptly been labelled therapeutic nihilism. Louis had won a victory, but it was dearly bought. What was lost was not only a number of useless or harmful treatments, but clinicians' interest in clinical research.[99]

Towards the end of the century a revival of critical clinical thinking was seen in Poland, and Bieganski discussed many of those topics that are also considered in this book, but this interesting intermezzo in the history of medicine was short-lived and had little international impact.[100,101]

The biostatistical approach to clinical medicine that had been introduced by Louis and Gavaret was almost forgotten for more than a century.

The era of laboratory research

The new development that originated in this vacuum proved more viable. Scientifically minded doctors realized that the time-honoured speculative disease theories had to be rejected, and that they would not be able to develop rational treatments unless they gained new knowledge about the pathogenesis of different diseases. Intellectually, they turned their backs on the everyday problems of clinical practice and retired to the newly established research laboratories.

Myxoedema was one of those diseases that attracted the interest of the medical scientists. It had been described as a disease entity in the 1870s, and a few years later Kocher and Reverdin from Switzerland observed the same clinical picture after thyroidectomy. In 1884 Schiff found that experimental myxoedema in dogs could be prevented by a previous thyroid graft, and this finding led Murray to treat myxoedema with injections of thyroid extract. Howitz of Copenhagen introduced peroral treatment in 1892 and myxoedema became the first disease to be fully controlled by pharmacotherapy. The example illustrates the interplay between clinical and laboratory research on an international scale which continues today. The later development need not to be discussed in detail. The introduction of insulin treatment of diabetes, treatment of pernicious anaemia with raw liver and later vitamin B_{12}, and treatment of infectious diseases with sulphonamides and penicillin are well-known milestones.

However, as Lasègue (1810–83) said about his laboratory-oriented colleagues,[1] 'They explain much or rather they explain everything and they pass quickly from hypothesis to practice'. Doctors have always had a tendency to overestimate their theoretical knowledge and that may easily lead to the introduction of ineffective or harmful treatments. They believe that they fully understand the pathogenesis of a disease and the mechanism of action of some treatment, but unfortunately the human organism is so complex that it is rarely possible to predict with certainty the effects of a new treatment. Only experience can show whether a treatment is more beneficial than harmful, and as long as that experience was uncontrolled, the situation remained much the same as in the pre-scientific era.

Anticoagulant treatment of myocardial infarction is a good example. In the 1950s the coagulation mechanisms of the blood attracted considerable interest.

The disease myocardial infarction was, in those days, called coronary thrombosis and it was considered rational to treat the patients with the newly discovered vitamin K antagonists. Papers were published where clinicians reported their excellent results and soon the treatment was accepted on both sides of the Atlantic. At that time randomized clinical trials (as described in Chapter 6) were still very rare, but when they were done 10 years later it was found that the treatment with vitamin K antagonists had no beneficial effect in this disease.

Oxygen treatment of chronic respiratory failure also illustrates that apparently rational treatments may be dangerous. Anybody with a little knowledge of respiratory physiology will realize that cyanosed and dyspnoeic patients suffer from hypoxia, but treatment with oxygen at high concentrations must have caused the death of thousands of patients until the danger of carbon dioxide narcosis was realized in the 1950s. At that time it was not possible to monitor the carbon dioxide concentration of arterial blood and it was only too easy to misinterpret the course of the clinical events. Imagine a cyanosed patient who is given too much oxygen. His colour improves almost immediately, his respiration is 'normalized', he falls asleep due to exhaustion and later he dies 'in spite of' the treatment.

The treatment of duodenal ulcer shows to what extent a generation of gastroenterologists were misled by uncontrolled experience. In the 1960s most patients were given a bland diet, an anticholinergic and an antacid whenever needed to relieve pain. Diet was the first of the treatments to be proved worthless, and in 1970 a carefully designed therapeutic trial showed that two commonly used anticholinergics had no appreciable clinical effect;[102] in a leading article in the *Lancet* they were aptly called 'logical placebos'.[103] Few clinicians, however, doubted the specific effect of antacids on ulcer pain, and it came as a surprise when is was found some years later that a potent liquid antacid was no better than a placebo preparation.[104] Then, for a time, no treatments were believed to be effective, until a new randomized trial showed that intensive antacid therapy, contrary to expectations, greatly enhanced ulcer healing.[105] Since then, of course, the introduction of new, more effective treatments has changed the picture.

Today we still use treatments that have not been adequately tested, and undoubtedly future generations of doctors will realize that some of them are totally useless. There is no reason to believe that our aptitude for drawing the right conclusions from clinical practice is any better than that of our predecessors. However, it remains to answer the question why clinicians throughout the history of medicine have been fooled by their uncontrolled experience and in order to do so it is necessary to consider four different factors: ignorance of the spontaneous course of the disease; regression towards the mean; runs of good or bad luck; and bias. It was previously believed that also the effect of placebo was important, but a recent systematic review (see Chapter 6) of all the randomized trials that had compared placebo tablets or other placebo interventions with no treatment found that it is doubtful whether placebos have a true, clinically relevant effect.[106,107]

The spontaneous course of the disease

Treatment of different diseases has always been standardized to a large extent, and doctors who always treat patients with the same disease in the same manner are bound to lose touch with the course of the disease when no treatment is given. Therefore, it is only to be expected that doctors, when treating diseases of short duration, sometimes mistake spontaneous recovery for an effect of their therapeutic efforts. In 1809, for instance, a doctor recommended belladonna as a remedy against whooping cough as 'the cough disappears after 6 or 8 weeks, occasionally earlier'.[108] Probably this observation was correct, but it should not be attributed to the treatment. Admittedly, it is easy in the daily routine to interpret simple coincidence as a causal relationship. When urinary tract infections are treated with sulphonamide and the symptoms subside within a few days, it is tempting to conclude that the treatment was effective, but quite often it is revealed that this was not the case. That happens when, in due time, the result of the urine culture arrives and it is disclosed that the bacteria were resistant to sulphonamide.

Similar misinterpretations find their way into even the best medical journals. Readers of reviews were informed in the British Medical Journal[109] and the Lancet[110] in 1994, and in New England Journal of Medicine[111] in 2001, that it was possible, using certain treatments, to stop bleeding in 'up to' 80–95% of patients with bleeding oesophageal varices. That suggests a huge treatment effect, but the authors failed to mention that the rate of spontaneous bleeding arrest can be very high in the untreated control groups of randomized trials.[112] Furthermore, clinicians need to know what the effect is, on average, and not in a selected series of patients with particularly successful outcomes.

It may also be difficult to judge correctly a treatment effect in chronic diseases. The severity of the symptoms in ulcerative colitis, bronchial asthma, rheumatoid arthritis and numerous other conditions fluctuate, as illustrated by Fig. 5.1, and clinicians may easily be deceived if they ignore this fact. Imagine a patient with ulcerative colitis who has been symptom-free for a long period of time and then suffers a relapse. After a while (at point a on the curve) she decides to see a doctor, who then refers her to a specialist. The severity of the

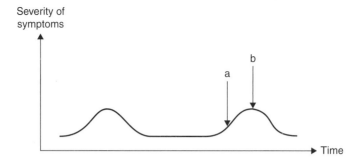

Fig. 5.1 Fluctuations of disease activity in a case of ulcerative colitis. a) The patient sees her doctor. b) The patient is referred to a specialist who starts a new treatment.

symptoms continues to increase until the specialist finds time to see her (at point b on the curve), but at that time she is on the verge of a spontaneous remission and any treatment will appear to be effective. Naturally, this course of events is by no means a certainty, but it may happen sufficiently often to make the specialist inform her colleagues that, according to her personal experience, the treatment used helps a considerable number of patients with ulcerative colitis.

Another example illustrates the same phenomenon particularly well. It was once believed that X-ray treatment was effective in osteoarthritis and spondylosis, and the patients were told that sometimes the effect would show immediately, sometimes it would only be evident after a few weeks, and sometimes the pain would get worse before the effect set in. This experience was useless, as it was the spontaneous fluctuations of the disease and not the treatment effect that was described. We should remember that patients tend to seek our advice when their symptoms are getting worse.

Regression towards the mean

The concept of regression towards the mean was introduced in Chapter 2. If we determine the serum cholesterol in a number of patients whose cholesterol level is completely normal, then we must expect, due to the imprecision (limited reproducibility) of the chemical analysis, that some of the results are high and others low. If we repeat the measurements some days later (still assuming that the patients' cholesterol levels are normal) we shall also obtain some high results and some low results, but probably not in the same patients. The cholesterol will seem to fall if initially it was high, and rise if it was low. This regularity is to be expected whenever we repeat the observation of a variable phenomenon. If we observe the flow of traffic, we shall probably find that a very large car is followed by a smaller car, and that a very small car is followed by a larger car. Galton reported in 1885 that tall parents usually had children who were shorter than themselves, whereas short parents usually had taller children.[113]

Regression towards the mean may simulate a treatment effect. If, for instance, the serum cholesterol is measured once in all patients with ischaemic heart disease, and treatment is instituted in all those with a high value, a decrease in the serum cholesterol will be recorded at the next visit in a number of cases, whether or not the treatment had any effect. That is to be expected due to analytic imprecision, but the phenomenon is further accentuated by the day-to-day variation of the patients' cholesterol levels. The same applies to blood pressure measurements where day-to-day variation may be caused both by the imprecision of the recording of the blood pressure and by fluctuations of the actual blood pressure. No doubt some patients have been treated unnecessarily for years because their doctor only measured their blood pressure once before treatment was instituted.

The apparent improvement of chronically ill patients with a fluctuating course, as described above, is one more example of regression towards the mean, due to the fact that clinicians usually see their patients when the symptoms are at their worst.

The interpretation of descriptive data may also be confounded by regression towards the mean if the reproducibility is not perfect, i.e. if kappa in inter- or intra-observer studies is less than one. If, for instance, a series of patients with ulcer symptoms are subjected to a duodenoscopy twice, the diagnoses may well differ, as it is possible to miss the ulcer and as the distinction between an erosion and a small ulcer is somewhat subjective. Sometimes an ulcer will be diagnosed the first time, but not the second time, and sometimes an ulcer will not be diagnosed the first time, but only the second time. Imagine then that a gastroenterologist treats only those patients with ulcer symptoms who are found to have an ulcer and subjects these to a repeat duodenoscopy a few weeks later. Even if no ulcers have healed, she will record that the ulcer has 'disappeared' in some patients and she may interpret this finding as a treatment effect. This is a common phenomenon. If the second assessment of the pulmonary scintigrams in the example in Chapter 2 (p. 24) had represented the assessment of a new set of scans after treatment for one month, one might have concluded that the cure rate was about 50% as the number of positive scintigrams had fallen from 22 to 11. The phenomenon is also bound to occur in randomized clinical trials, where it may explain some of the 'cures' in untreated control groups.

Run of luck

Clinicians' personal experience is often limited to a relatively small number of cases and they may easily be deceived by a run of good or bad luck. It is encouraging if 40 out of 50 patients (80%) are cured by a new surgical operation, especially if the prognosis without surgery is known to be very poor, but it is necessary to ask the question to which extent such limited experience is reliable.

This is a statistical problem that may be illustrated by a simple model. We may imagine a chest of drawers filled with a very large number of black and white marbles. These marbles symbolize all present and future patients with the disease in question, i.e. the hypothetical population of patients. The white marbles represent those patients who are cured by the operation, whereas the black marbles represent those who die. The percentage of white and black marbles in the chest is unknown.

From this chest we sample 50 marbles at random, and we find that 40 are white and 10 are black. Then the question is asked: What can we conclude from this sample as regards the true percentage of white marbles in the chest?

Common sense tells us that it is very unlikely that the true percentage is, say, 10%, because we do not expect chance to cheat us that much. We can handle this problem by using statistical calculations. We can calculate the probability of obtaining our result given any percentage of white marbles in the chest, and, by means of such calculations, we can say within what limits the true percentage may be expected to lie. In this case, using the conventional statistical terminology, we will find that the lower and upper limits of the 95% confidence interval are 66.3% and 90.0%.

It is easiest to explain the concept of confidence intervals by making a distinction between rare and common events and by defining rare events as those that occur less than 5% of the time. Using this definition, the calculation has shown that the observed cure rate of 80% would have been a rare event if the true cure rate was lower than the lower confidence limit or larger than the upper confidence limit. When we calculate the 95% confidence interval we shall, in the long run, be right 19 out of 20 times when we make the assumption that the interval includes the true value.

It does not follow from this argument, however, that we should feel 95% confident that the confidence interval in a particular study includes the true value. Imagine, for instance, that we do a thorough search of the literature, which reveals that other surgeons who did the same operation on average only cured 60% of their patients. Then we must seriously consider the possibility that the results obtained by this surgeon only represented a run of good luck. In other words, we should no longer be almost sure, i.e. 95% confident, that the true cure rate fell within the interval. We should have to consider the possibility that her result was one of the rare events where the true value falls outside the interval.

Fig. 5.2 illustrates the expected variation of the results, if the true cure rate were exactly 60%, and if 40 equally proficient surgeons, independently of one another, had done a series of 50 operations on similar patients. The observed cure rate and the 95% confidence interval are shown for each of these series, and it is seen that in most cases the interval includes the true cure rate of 60%. In one series (A), however, the true cure rate exceeds the upper confidence limit, and in another (B) it is lower than the lower confidence limit.

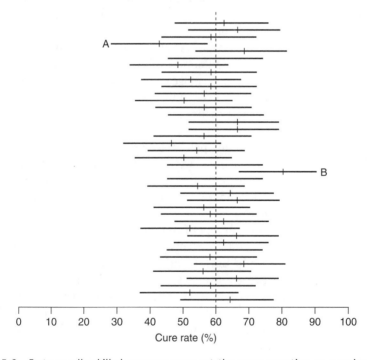

Fig. 5.2 Forty equally skilled surgeons carry out the same operation on a series of 50 patients each. It is assumed that the true cure rate is 60%. The figure shows the observed cure rate (with 95% confidence interval) for each series.

If the true cure rate was, in fact, 60%, our surgeon's result would correspond to the series marked B, but we cannot exclude the alternative explanation that she is, in fact, more skilled than her colleagues and that the true cure rate in her case is higher. To prove this she would have to do the operation on many more patients.

The distinction between frequential (statistical) and subjective probabilities, which was introduced in Chapter 4, is important in this context. Statisticians concern themselves with frequential probabilities; they tell us that in the long run we shall be right 19 out of 20 times when we make the assumption that the true value falls within the 95% confidence interval. Readers of medical journals, on the other hand, wish to assess the subjective probability of (their confidence in) the assumption that the interval includes the true value in a particular study, and that assessment is based not only on the results of that study, but also on other kinds of information, such as the results of other studies or, in this case, additional information about the surgeon. We should, for instance, feel more confident that she is doing better than her colleagues, if she also has a reputation of being more deft than others when she does other types of surgical operations. Therefore, the expression, 95% confidence interval, applies to groups of patients, but does not tell us how confident we should be in an individual case.

It follows that confidence intervals must always be interpreted with care, but nonetheless they are of fundamental importance in the context of evidence-based medicine, both when we assess our own clinical experience critically and when we assess the results of others from articles in medical journals. The exact figures reported in the journals only refer to those patients who were observed by the author, and we need to assess to what extent those results can be extrapolated to other patients, especially our own. The determination of confidence intervals serves this important purpose.

The width of the confidence interval depends on the number of patients, which is only to be expected as greater experience allows more precise predictions (see an approximated formula on p. 134). If the surgeon had observed that 8 out of 10 patients were cured, the interval would have been 44.4% to 97.5%, and, if she had observed that 80 out of 100 were cured, the interval would have been 70.8% to 87.3%.

Bias

Regression towards the mean and runs of good or bad luck illustrate the influence of random errors, but uncontrolled clinical experience may also be distorted by systematic errors (bias).

Previously, clinicians often published the results they had obtained by treating a series of patients, but the scientific value of such studies was very small. Usually, the diagnostic criteria, the indications for using the treatment and the criteria for assessing the effects were not defined in advance, and in that case there are numerous sources of bias. Possibly, the severely ill (or mildly ill) patients were not included, and possibly, the final diagnosis, which determined the inclusion in the series, was influenced by the treatment result. In general, little attention should be paid to such studies, which are not prospective and which have not been carried out according to a detailed protocol.

Even well-planned studies of the effect of some treatment are of little use if there is no control group, except perhaps in the context of quality assurance. If, for instance, the outcome of a particular surgical operation varies in different surgical departments, one should, of course, explore the possible reasons for that variation.

The reliability of uncontrolled series of treatment results is particularly low, if the results have been recorded nowhere but in the memory of the physician, as those cases which took an unusual course stick in the mind much more easily than the others. If we ask a colleague to tell us about the effect of a particular treatment, she will be inclined to overestimate the benefits if some patients fared surprisingly well, and she may warn us against the treatment, if a few patients fared surprisingly badly. This phenomenon is called *recall bias*, and the exceptional cases may very well have an undue influence on the treatment of future patients. Once a single case of cerebral haemorrhage due to anticoagulant treatment made a clinician refrain from using that treatment even when it was clearly indicated.

Optimism bias[114] is also important. Clinicians hope that their patients get better and that their treatments are successful. That is of course a laudable attitude, but it also has the effect that clinicians are biased observers. They convince themselves that the patients look a little better or that the symptoms are a little less severe. This optimism may create a psychological game between doctor and patient with the result that the patient, too, says that she feels a little better either because she believes so or because she wishes to please the doctor.

The placebo effect

The word *placebo* means 'I shall please' and it was first used in the context of medical treatment towards the end of the eighteenth century. In Motherby's *New Medical Dictionary* from 1785 placebo is defined as 'a commonplace method or medicine calculated to amuse for a time, rather than for any other purpose'.[2]

Since then expressions like placebo, placebo phenomenon, placebo treatment and placebo effect have gained use both within and without the medical profession, also when no allusion is made to the therapist's intentions, and confusion reigns. Much has been written about this topic, but no generally accepted stringent definition exists[115,116] and it may be impossible to define placebo in a way that avoids logical inconsistencies.[117] According to common language usage, however, the placebo effect is the therapeutic effect of the treatment setting as a whole, including the doctor–patient relationship, i.e. a beneficial effect that cannot (yet?) be explained by physiological and metabolic processes. The alleged effect may be increased well-being, alleviation of specific symptoms (typically pain), normalization of objective findings or the prevention of disease or disease complications. One may also talk about a 'negative' placebo effect or a nocebo effect (derived from Latin *nocere* = harm), if the patient's condition gets worse.

Clinicians often report that they observed a beneficial effect of the prescription of a drug, which they themselves regarded as completely ineffective. If the drug was given as tablets, they may even use the term 'placebo tablets', but taken literally that is misleading, as it is not implied that the tablets themselves have a mysterious effect. It is the prescription of the tablets that is believed to be effective, and it is not suggested that they would have had a similar effect, if, for instance, they had been given to a laboratory animal or if the patient had found them in the street. It is also believed that the placebo phenomenon may play an important role when clinicians prescribe drugs with a well-established specific effect (i.e. antirheumatic drugs which inhibit the synthesis of prostaglandins in both humans and animals), as the observed treatment result may then be regarded as the sum of the specific effect and the placebo effect.

The analysis of the placebo concept raises two kinds of questions, firstly ontological questions, i.e. questions about the true nature of the phenomenon, and empirical questions, i.e. questions concerning the demonstration of the phenomenon by means of clinical research.

It is usually assumed that the placebo effect is mediated via a purely psychological or psychosomatic mechanism. The concept of psychosomatic mechanisms is disputed, but if we accept that the sensation of fear may cause adrenalin release, a rise in blood pressure and palpitations, it is not such a mysterious idea that other subjective experiences could have a beneficial effect. Psychosomatic theory is related to those philosophical body–mind theories, according to which mental phenomena such as anxiety, hunger, pain and even negative and positive expectations may cause bodily phenomena. However, some philosophers, e.g. behaviourists, would dispute that.[13]

It has been asserted that some phenomena that are usually regarded as placebo effects can be explained within conventional physiological theory. For example, it has been suggested that a possible pain reducing effect of injection of saline or of acupuncture is caused by the release of endorphins, but a critical review of the relevant studies concluded that this hypothesis has not been convincingly documented.[118] It should also be noted that if the explanation were true, there would be no good reason to call the effect a placebo effect.[117]

These speculations about the true nature of the placebo phenomenon do not tell us how to demonstrate and measure possible placebo effects. Most of the studies, which are quoted again and again by those who emphasize the great significance of the placebo phenomenon, are simply observations on series of patients who received a treatment that was considered pharmacologically inactive. It is, for instance, often mentioned that placebo treatment relieves headache. The headache likely disappears after a while, but the spontaneous course of an attack of headache was not taken into account. This kind of 'proof' made Beecher conclude in a much quoted paper that in various conditions the placebo effect is 35%, on average.[119]

The introduction of the randomized clinical trial stimulated interest in the placebo phenomenon, which was then regarded as a source of error which might confound the interpretation of the results. Blinded studies were recommended where the patients in the control group received inactive tablets, e.g. lactose tablets. Unfortunately, these tablets are often called placebo tablets, just as the control group is called the placebo group, and the effect observed in the control group is called the placebo effect. Using this terminology, the placebo effect in duodenal ulcer trials may be said to vary between 30% and 60%, as the healing rates in the control groups are of this order of magnitude. It cannot, of course, be excluded that the patients' expectations may promote ulcer healing, but the observed effect among the controls can easily be explained by a combination of spontaneous healing and, as explained above, regression towards the mean due to observer variation at endoscopy.

About 50 years after Beecher's article a systematic review (see Chapter 6) was published of 130 randomized trials that all compared a patient group that received a placebo intervention with a group that was not treated.[106] This review, which has subsequently been updated with more trials,[107] could not detect any effect of placebo on objective outcomes. There was apparently a minor effect on subjective outcomes, corresponding to only 6.5 mm on a 100 mm visual analogue scale for pain, but this result could be caused by bias.

It is not possible to blind trials where half of the patients do not receive any treatment and the other half receive treatment with a placebo.

There are also trials where two groups of patients have received the same treatment under different circumstances, but most have methodological flaws.[118] A Dutch group that reviewed hundreds of articles only recovered four that they thought were acceptable.[120] I will mention two such studies. One, much quoted, randomized trial suggested that the physician's attitude and the information given to the patient could be important.[121] A general practitioner included 200 patients with nonspecific symptoms and allocated them, at random, to four groups: positive or negative consultations with or without treatment. At the positive consultations the patients received a 'fake diagnosis' and were informed that they would soon feel much better. They were either told that no treatment was needed, or they were given inactive tablets with the information that they would have a good effect. At the negative consultations the clinician told the patients that he did not know what was wrong and that therefore he could prescribe no treatment, or he prescribed inactive tablets with the additional information that it was not certain that they would have any effect. Improvement was recorded in 64 of those 100 patients who received a positive consultation, and only in 39 of 100 patients who received a negative consultation; the prescription of inactive tablets seemed to make no difference. This trial, of course, presents considerable ethical and methodological problems, but I shall not discuss these here. More importantly, other researchers that tried to replicate this result in a similar trial did not find an effect of a positive consultation.[122]

We will need to accept that it has not been demonstrated convincingly that a placebo intervention can have an effect on the course of the disease. On the other hand there is little doubt that the clinician's attitude, her confidence in the prescribed treatment and the information given to the patients may influence the way in which they perceive their symptoms and their general condition. The technical term, a placebo effect, which cannot even be defined in a consistent way, should therefore be abandoned. It is only to be expected that patients who worry about some subjective symptom will feel relieved when they hear that it is not serious. This was true of a colleague who once developed pain in the chest irradiating to the left arm; he was naturally worried, but when the typical vesicular eruption of herpes zoster appeared, the pain bothered him no longer. Such experiences indicate that one should interpret the results of patient surveys very cautiously. Those patients who had a fear of serious disease disproved will tend to see everything in a positive light, whereas those who had their suspicion confirmed will tend to be less satisfied with their hospital stay.

Other randomized trials show more tangible effects of the clinical setting. It has, for instance, been reported that the presence of a person providing continuous support to women during childbirth had the effect that the women were more likely to have a spontaneous vaginal birth, and less likely to have intrapartum analgesia or to report dissatisfaction with their childbirth experiences.[123] It is not easy to interpret these results, however. It could be that the feeling of security induced by the continuous presence of a supportive person makes it easier for the woman to accept the inconveniences of childbirth, or that it merely keeps the clinicians away from interfering with natural childbirths.

It is sometimes argued by doctors who give great credence to the placebo phenomenon that it may be justified to prescribe inactive treatments and to suggest to the patient, either implicitly or explicitly, that the treatment is effective. This practice is quite unacceptable from an ethical point of view, as it is hard to conceive that any patient seeking medical assistance expects to be wilfully deceived. However, recognition of the importance of security, understanding and trust may induce clinicians to pay greater attention to the human aspects of the doctor–patient relationship. It is very likely that a clinician who shows a genuine interest in the patient's situation and takes the necessary time to explain the results of investigations and the nature of the patient's disease will get more satisfied patients than the colleague who prescribes inactive tablets.

The need for controlled experience

Uncontrolled experience cannot be trusted and therefore it is necessary to test new treatments by means of controlled trials, i.e. trials where the effect of the new treatment is compared with the effect of the standard treatment or no treatment at all. This can be done in a number of ways.

One may simply introduce the new treatment in the daily routine and record the treatment result in a series of patients. Then these results are compared with those that were obtained in a series of historical controls, i.e. patients who during a preceding period received the old treatment. This procedure, however, cannot be recommended. Usually, the historical data are retrieved from the patients' notes, which are rarely sufficiently reliable to serve scientific purposes, but there are other sources of error. The adjuvant treatment may have been improved from the first period to the next, or the diagnostic methods may have been refined with the result that those patients who received the new treatment were less severely ill than those who received the old treatment. That was probably one of the reasons why the introduction of anticoagulant therapy in the 1950s was accompanied by a fall in the fatality rate of myocardial infarction. Studies of this kind will also be biased, if the clinicians refrain from treating severely ill patients with a new experimental treatment, while such patients were not excluded from the historical controls.[124] Although this is common knowledge, oncologists often take all the credit for the improved survival of cancer patients (measured from time of diagnosis) as they, undoubtedly for a political gain, choose to disregard the fact that the diagnosis is often made several years earlier in the course of the disease today than it was decades ago.[51]

As an alternative one may introduce the new treatment at one hospital and continue using the old one at another hospital. That method, however, is also seriously unreliable, as we would not expect the patients to be fully comparable or the adjuvant therapy to be identical.

Fibiger had realized these problems when he published the results of a controlled trial of the effect of an antitoxin in diphtheria during childhood in 1898.[125,126] Four hundred and eighty-four children entered the trial, which lasted for one year, serum treatment and no treatment being given on alternate days. He observed eight deaths in the treatment group compared with 30 deaths in the equally large control group. The methods may not have been perfect according to present-day standards, but the trial was unique in an international context, and Fibiger was far ahead of his time.

The breakthrough only occurred after the Second World War when the Medical Research Council promoted the use of randomized clinical trials. By recommending random allocation of the patients to the different treatment groups, the reliability of the results was greatly enhanced. The streptomycin trial of pulmonary tuberculosis which was initiated by, among others, Bradford Hill, was started in 1946 and the positive results were published two years later.[127] The negative results of new treatments, which had initially been accepted uncritically, such as anticoagulant treatment of myocardial infarction and anticholinergic treatment of peptic ulcers, as well as the detection of thousands of newborns with serious birth defects in the 1960s caused by thalidomide,[128] also paved the way for general acceptance of randomized trials. The methods used today will be explained in the next chapter.

Alternative medicine: pseudoscientific thinking

This historical account might leave the impression that 'pseudoscientific' reasoning is now a thing of the past, and that at long last we have accepted that uncontrolled experience cannot be trusted and that all new treatments must be subjected to well-planned randomized trials. That, however, is not the case.

Alternative medicine is flourishing, and it is as if many patients and some doctors are actually attracted by its irrationality.

Here I shall not discuss all the bizarre offers of the alternative market, but there is much to choose between. Diagnoses are made by inspecting the patient's iris, by examining the patient's aura or by recording the propagation of the vibrations from a tuning fork placed on the knee. A large variety of herbs and special minerals are given as treatments, and so is application of magnetic or psychic force, the latter sometimes even at a distance. We encounter theories that superficially mimic scientific ones, and others that are associated with Eastern mysticism. I shall only mention a few of the more well-established schools and will use the collective term alternative medicine although others prefer to talk about nonconventional or complementary medicine.[129]

Homoeopathy was founded by Samuel Hahnemann towards the end of the eighteenth century. He developed the doctrine that 'like is cured by like', which is rooted in medieval medicine, and according to which patients presenting certain symptoms must be treated with those drugs which in healthy persons elicit similar symptoms. Thus, Hahnemann argued that in healthy persons quinine may provoke the symptoms of malaria and that therefore it acts curatively in that disease. A second doctrine is even more peculiar. It is held that infinitesimally small doses must be used, meaning that the preparation may be diluted so much that it is not certain that the patient ingests one single molecule. Homoeopaths are fully aware of this fact but believe that the preparation has left some sort of imprint in the solvent.[130] Homoeopathy has never been very popular in Scandinavia, but thousands of homoeopaths practice in, for instance, Great Britain, the United States and Germany.

Chiropractic is also a well-established school. It was founded in 1895 by Palmer, an American magnetic healer, and he believed that all diseases, including peptic ulcers, hypertension, diabetes, epilepsy, cancer and infections were caused by small vertebral misalignments called subluxations.[131] Consequently, chiropractic therapy involves the detection and correction of these misalignments by means of manual manipulations, so-called 'adjustments'. Palmer's son treated infections with manipulations, and a little time spent surfing the Internet shows that chiropractic treatment is still used in children's asthma, hay fever, otitis and nocturnal enuresis. Some chiropractors claim that they confine themselves to the treatment of musculoskeletal diseases and that they accept the tradition of the natural sciences, but if they give up the idea of the pathogenic role of subluxations it is difficult to see the difference between chiropractic and physical medicine. A large randomized trial of chiropractic treatment of patients with back pain showed only a marginal effect,[132] and systematic reviews of such trials have not been encouraging either.[133]

I shall also briefly mention reflexology, especially reflex zone therapy of the feet, which originated in the East and which has become very popular in some countries. It is believed that localized reflex points on the sole of the foot are connected with different parts of the body, and charts have been drawn showing the position of these points. Pressure applied on the right point is said to have a healing effect on the corresponding organ, be it the kidneys, the gall bladder or perhaps the heart. Needless to say, these speculations have not been documented in clinical studies.

Since 1964 an American magician, James Randi, has offered a one-million-dollar prize to anyone who, under controlled observing conditions, can show evidence that pseudoscientific claims are correct, for example the alleged mechanism of action for the effect of homoeopathy, chiropractic healing (apart from back and joint problems) and reflexology.[134] Many have tried but none have succeeded.

When alternative therapists are asked why they believe that their treatments are effective, they will usually refer to their own personal experience and in some cases they may add that their treatment has ancient roots and that it would have been abandoned centuries ago, if it were ineffective. These arguments are obviously invalid. I have already discussed in some detail the fallacies of uncontrolled experience, and ineffective treatments that originated in Greek Antiquity were used in Europe as late as the nineteenth century.

Many proponents of alternative practices also claim that their theories are holistic, i.e. take into account both the bodily and the spiritual aspects of the nature of man, whereas scientific medicine is reductionistic, i.e. reduces man to a biological organism and endeavours to explain disease in physicochemical terms. These are difficult philosophical concepts, but in this context the use of the words seems mainly rhetorical. It is, for instance, difficult to imagine anything more 'reductionistic' than the theory that all kinds of diseases are caused by subluxations in the vertebral column. Nor does the idea that a wide spectrum of very different ailments can be cured by the intake of one particular mineral or by rubbing the soles of the feet seem particularly 'holistic'. It is, of course, to some extent true that medical science is reductionistic, but the clinician who seeks the physiological cause of the patient's symptoms need not – indeed should not – ignore the ethical and hermeneutic aspects of the decision process (see Chapter 7). Holism is a vague concept, and as yet no alternative school has suggested a credible theory that explains the age-old body–mind problem.

Any discussion of the fundamental difference between alternative and scientific medicine presupposes that these terms have been defined, and that is not easy. Members of the medical profession debating this question, often leave the impression that scientific medicine, almost by definition, is that which is practised by authorized medical doctors whereas alternative medicine is that which is practised by others. But this distinction is not tenable, as it is difficult to claim that medical doctors always reason scientifically and as some of them prescribe alternative medicine. Homoeopathic therapy does not become scientific because it is used by an ill-advised medical doctor.

It is also unreasonable to claim that the theories of alternative medicine are always wrong, and that those of scientific medicine are always true. Admittedly, most alternative theories are so much at variance with our knowledge of physics, chemistry and physiology that they must be regarded as false, but the theories of scientific medicine are not invulnerable. Many of the theories found in the standard textbooks today will some time in the future be modified or rejected.

One might also suggest that alternative therapeutic practices are ineffective, whereas those treatments that are used by medical doctors are effective. This distinction is obviously unacceptable as medical practitioners use many ineffective treatments, and as some alternative treatments have considerable effects. Herbal drugs sold as 'natural medicines' sometimes contain active substances with, for instance, antipyretic, anticholinergic or laxative effects and these effects are, of course, noticed by the patients. It is, however, difficult to see that it should be more 'natural' to take such drugs with an unknown content of a variety of substances, rather than taking an exact amount of a well-defined drug. In fact, such drugs can be dangerous. Many herbal creams have been adulterated with an undeclared content of corticosteroids in therapeutic amounts,[135] and fatal illness has been reported after the intake of Chinese herbal tea.[136]

The main difference between alternative and scientific medicine is rather more subtle; it reflects the difference between scientific and pseudoscientific thinking. Scientific thinking is characterized by a critical attitude to established theories on the part of the scientists. They seek weak points in the theories, generate new hypotheses and subject these to critical experiments. According to Popper, we must accept that our scientific theories are only approximations to the truth, and their trustworthiness depends on the zeal with which they have been exposed to critical experiments.[137]

The proponents of alternative medicine do not reason like that. Reflexologists, for instance, do not test whether they have charted the position of the reflex points on the sole of the foot correctly, e.g. whether it makes any difference to patients with gall bladder disease if the pressure is applied to the 'kidney point' or vice versa, and homoeopaths do not expose their theory of 'like is cured by like' to critical experiments. One proponent of homoeopathy even argued that it was one of the strengths of homoeopathy that it was the same today as in Hahneman's days, whereas medical theories change all the time. The homoeopaths had found the truth.[130]

Some alternative practitioners argue that it is not possible to study their treatments in randomized trials, because the trial setting is artificial and will decrease the effect. However, empirical studies do not suggest that this is important,[138] and it is now broadly accepted that alternative treatments must be tested in randomized trials. This has also occurred. Many randomized trials have compared a homoeopathic treatment with no treatment, and a systematic review revealed a general trend in favour of 'active' treatment.[139] This is an interesting review, but only because it reveals the importance of bias (I shall write more about this review in the next chapter).

Even results from randomized trials should be interpreted with great caution if the underlying theory is obviously absurd, like for homoeopathy. Carrying out randomized trials must in this case be regarded as a somewhat futile exercise, as the acceptance of a result in favour of the treatment always requires a modicum of prior belief. Surprisingly, in 2006, the Medicines and Healthcare Products Agency in the UK allowed manufacturers of homoeopathic products to specify the ailments they could be used for.[140] The health minister argued that homoeopathic products are different from conventional medicines and cannot demonstrate efficacy in the same way that conventional medicinal products are required to do to. Needless to say, this double standard in drug regulation caused a public outcry from scientists and doctors.

It is also a controversial issue whether or not acupuncture has a clinically relevant effect on pain. Hundreds of trials and many systematic reviews have been carried out with acupuncture,[141] but the methodological quality of the trials is generally low and in the best trials, acupuncture was quite often no better than placebo acupuncture. Should an effect be demonstrated convincingly in the future, this would not prove, of course, that the ancient Chinese theory of the twelve meridians is true, as it is possible to draw true conclusions from false premises.

In short, alternative medicine brings to mind the state of clinical medicine in the eighteenth century when the age-old theory of the four humours and a variety of new, equally speculative theories of disease were flourishing. In those days medical practitioners, just like the proponents of alternative medicine today, believed that their uncontrolled experience confirmed the figments of their imagination. Alternative treatments are an anachronism in modern therapeutics.

6

The Randomized Clinical Trial

Comparative experience is a prerequisite for experimental and scientific medicine, otherwise the physician may walk at random and become the sport of a thousand illusions.

Claude Bernard[142]

The half-life of medical knowledge is short and it is difficult for medical practitioners to keep up-to-date. The medical journals regularly publish the results of clinical trials that suggest that some new treatment is better than the current one, and then it is not enough to read the abstract with the author's conclusions. The perfect scientific investigation has yet to be seen, and the critical reader must be well acquainted with the methodological pitfalls of clinical research.

The randomized clinical trial is the gold standard for the assessment of any intervention, not only pharmacotherapy, but also surgical interventions, physiotherapy, dietary treatment, different types of nursing care, preventive measures in the general population, and, as I have discussed in Chapter 4 (p. 85), also for assessment of the value of diagnostic tests. In this chapter I shall explain what basic knowledge clinicians ought to have when they study a trial report. Those who wish to do such trials themselves must seek additional information elsewhere.[9,143]

Very often a standard design is used. A number of patients with the disease in question are allocated at random to two groups, the treatment group and the control group. The patients in the treatment group receive the new treatment, whereas those in the control group typically receive the treatment in current use.

If possible, the trial is blinded, which implies that patients and investigators, and sometimes other people involved with the trial, do not know to which group the individual patient belongs. The results of the two treatments are recorded and subjected to a statistical analysis. We shall now consider this design step by step.

Selection of patients

The 'Methods' section of the report of a randomized trial is sometimes written in small print, but it deserves special attention. The reader wishes to assess if he can use the results for the benefit of his own patients, and the included patients should therefore be described in some detail to enable the reader to judge whether they are sufficiently similar to his patients.

The entry criteria (e.g. diagnostic criteria, severity of the disease and para-clinical findings) and exclusion criteria (e.g. pregnancy and concomitant disease) should be so well defined that the reader can recognize the patients. Occasionally, the report only provides the information that a certain number of patients diagnosed after standard criteria with, say, asthma, an irritable bowel syndrome or myocardial infarction were included, and such trials are of limited value, as different clinicians use different diagnostic criteria for the diagnosis of these diseases.

Ideally, all patients fulfilling the entry criteria during the period of the trial should be enrolled, but that can rarely be achieved. It is, for instance, necessary to obtain the patients' informed consent, and some patients will probably refuse to take part. If, however, many patients fail to be included, the remainder may no longer constitute a representative sample of all patients fulfilling the entry criteria. The possible effect of such *sampling bias* for the outcome of the trial depends on the clinical problem, and sometimes it cannot be ignored. If, for instance, only 30% of those women with breast cancer who fulfilled the entry criteria had accepted participation in one of those trials that compared radical mastectomy and tumorectomy, it might have been difficult to interpret the results. Perhaps women with palpable tumours refused to participate as they feared that the new treatment, tumorectomy, might not be as good as the old one, or perhaps those with a small non-palpable tumour demonstrated by mammography did not want to lose their breast.

There is no perfect solution to this problem, apart from doing a subgroup analysis after the completion of the trial, comparing the treatment results in patients with palpable and non-palpable tumours. If the results were the same, the importance of this particular factor would have been disproved. For these reasons it can be useful if reports of randomized trials contain information about eligible patients who were not enrolled, permitting the reader to judge for himself whether or not sampling bias may have occurred.

Unfortunately, many trials are designed in such a way that it introduces serious sampling bias. Industry-sponsored drug trials routinely exclude patients above 65 years of age[144] even when most patients who will subsequently use the drug will be elderly. As an example, one study showed that those patients who received the antirheumatic drug, rofecoxib, in clinical practice had eight times higher risk of myocardial infarction than those patients who had been entered in the company's clinical trials.[145] It therefore took much longer than necessary before it became known that this drug causes thromboses at an unacceptably high rate.

As this example illustrates, the reader must carefully consider to what extent his own patients resemble those of the trial. A general practitioner cannot take it for granted that he will obtain the same results as specialists at teaching hospitals, as his patients belong to a different part of the clinical spectrum. An antidepressant that has been tested at a psychiatric hospital unit may not be equally effective in other settings. The diagnostic criteria may also be quite different. Patients with upper dyspepsia in general practice are obviously not the same as patients in a specialist practice with an endoscopically diagnosed duodenal ulcer. Geographical differences must also be taken into account. The frequency and manifestations of gastric cancer, for instance, are different in Japan compared with most European countries, and it cannot be excluded that the disease in these two parts of the world will respond differently to some new chemotherapy.

Randomization

As mentioned in the preceding chapter it is not sufficient to compare the results of a new treatment with those obtained previously or with those obtained at a different hospital, and unfortunately it cannot be recommended to let the patients themselves choose the treatment that they prefer. That suggestion was once made in connection with the breast cancer trials, but, for the reasons mentioned above, women with palpable cancers might have preferred mastectomy while those with non-palpable ones might have chosen a tumorectomy. It would have been impossible to interpret the results.

The only solution to these difficulties is *randomization*. Random allocation to the two treatment groups effectively prevents systematic differences, but, of course, imbalances may still occur due to random variation. If the number of patients is small, it cannot be excluded that patients who for some reason or other have a poor prognosis, simply by chance, predominate in one of the treatment groups, but, if the sample is sufficiently large, different types of patients will tend to be evenly distributed in the two groups. However, imbalances arising at random are subject to the laws of chance, and a proper statistical analysis will tell to which extent they may have influenced the results of the trial.

The randomization procedure is best explained by describing the method which was used prior to the introduction of computer technology and which is still sometimes used. At the planning stage a helper, who afterwards is not involved with the trial, produces the randomization sequence. If the sample size calculation[9] has shown that 120 patients are needed, the helper may, in principle, toss a coin 120 times (having decided in advance that 'heads' = treatment A and 'tails' = treatment B) and write down the sequence, e.g. AABABBBAABABAAB... In practice, however, he will simulate the tosses, using random number tables or series of random numbers generated by a computer. Then the clinician running the trial, who of course does not see the list, receives a stack of 120 firmly closed, opaque, numbered envelopes, each containing a card marked treatment A or treatment B.

If it is a blinded trial, which compares two drugs in tablet form, the clinician will also receive 120 numbered bottles, containing the right sort of tablets for each patient. In this case, an envelope will only be opened if the clinician needs to break the code because a serious harm occurred.

If the trial is not blinded, e.g. a trial comparing a medical and a surgical treatment, the clinician must of course open the numbered envelopes in succession each time a new patient enters the trial, in order to see which treatment to give.

This procedure is not foolproof if somebody wants to cheat. It may be possible to read what is written on the card if the envelope is held up to a bright light, and, if the trial is not blinded and several patients are admitted on the same day, it is possible to open several envelopes at once and then decide which patient should have which treatment.

Therefore, randomization by computer is now the standard procedure. The clinical investigator enters the entry criteria, and if (and only if) these are fulfilled the computer program will allocate the patient at random to one of the treatment groups and will then tell the investigator which treatment to use. This method is called *concealed allocation* because the clinician cannot know which treatment the patient will get before the patient has entered the trial with certainty.

Sometimes more elaborate randomization procedures are used in order to ensure that subgroups of patients are equally distributed in the two treatment groups. In large multicentre trials where each centre is expected to recruit, say, 10 patients, it may be useful to use *block randomization*, e.g. to randomize in blocks of 10, so that each centre provides 5 patients for the treatment group and 5 patients for the control group. One may also use randomization procedures that ensure that the two patient groups are comparable as regards severity of disease, length of history or some other factor of known or assumed prognostic significance. However, such prior subdivision or *stratification* of the patients makes a trial less easy to handle.

In the past more simple procedures were used. Sometimes the patients were allocated to the two treatments according to their date of birth (e.g. even date = new treatment and odd date = old treatment) or date of admission, but experience shows that the results of such trials must be interpreted with great caution. In one trial, which compared a surgical and a medical treatment, it was found afterwards that the average age of the surgically treated patients was lower than that of the medically treated ones. All patients who are considered bad risks from a surgical point of view, including those who are old and frail, must of course be excluded from a trial of this kind and, possibly, this exclusion criterion was treated more leniently among those who, according to their date of birth, were to receive medical treatment than among those who were to be treated surgically. Such bias can only be avoided if the following rule is applied: first it is decided whether the patient is eligible for the trial by fulfilling all the entry criteria, next it is determined by some random procedure which treatment the patient should be given, and finally it is ensured that entered patients cannot later 'disappear', which is best done by recording the entry data and the treatment allocation with a computer program that does not allow later changes to these data.

Randomization is the most important safeguard against bias in medical research. It should therefore be used whenever possible, e.g. also in animal experiments. And authors of journal articles should report what they did in detail, particularly as it has been shown that trials with inadequate randomization, or in which the randomization method was not described, tend to exaggerate the effect of a new treatment by about 20%, on average.[146] This is rather serious, as many of our treatments have an apparent effect of this magnitude. We may therefore assume that some of them, in reality, have no effect.

Choice of treatment in the control group

The patients in the experimental group receive the new treatment while those in the control group should, as a general rule, receive the one in current use.

Obviously, this is the right procedure from the point of view of the clinician who wishes to know whether or not the new treatment is any better than the standard treatment. He would not wish to change to the new treatment unless it is more effective, except perhaps in those relatively rare cases where it is cheaper or has fewer harms.

Alternatively, one may compare the new treatment with no treatment, which means that the patients in the control group of a blinded drug trial receive inert, dummy tablets. This design, however, is only acceptable from a clinical and an ethical point of view if no other effective treatment is available, in which case one may say that no treatment is the best current treatment. This is an important point as much of the criticism that has been raised against this type of research stems from the misconception that half the participating patients always receive inert tablets ('placebo tablets').

Representatives of the drug industry may, of course, take a different view of the matter. If they wish to register a new drug, they only have to prove that it is effective. Therefore, from their point of view it is sufficient to compare with inert tablets. They may also pay attention to the fact that a comparison of two effective drugs requires many more patients than a comparison with inert tablets. Such commercial interests are irrelevant from a clinical point of view, however.

Principles of blinding

Trials where the doctor as well as the patient knows which treatment is given, involve a considerable risk of bias. The doctor may be biased, having made up his mind in advance that the new treatment is best, and this belief may well influence the way in which he questions the patient and interprets the treatment result. The patients may also be biased as those who know that they are trying something new may have greater confidence in the effect than those who get the standard treatment. Studies have shown that trials that are not blinded tend to exaggerate the effect of a new treatment by about 14%, on average.[146] Unblinded trials are sometimes described as 'open-label', but this term should be abandoned as it can also mean a study without a control group.

Psychological bias can be reduced by blinding patients and clinicians. Most often, such trials are called double-blind, but this term, as well as the term single-blind, should also be abandoned, as investigators interpret them very differently.[147,148] Several other types of people may be involved with a trial, e.g. data collectors, data assessors, data analysts and manuscript writers, and all of these can also be blinded.[149] It is therefore necessary to describe in detail what measures were taken to obtain blinding and which types of people were intended to be blinded.

Blinding has other important advantages. If, for instance, some patients develop unexpected symptoms or signs, such as severe dizziness or an increase in liver enzymes, it is necessary to decide whether or not they should be withdrawn from the trial, and this decision may be biased if the trial is not blinded. The clinician may decide to withdraw a patient on the suspicion of an unknown harm if he receives the new treatment, but ignore the observation if he receives the standard treatment. As a result there would be more withdrawals due to suspected harms in the treatment group than in the control group. This problem does not arise in blinded trials where the clinician is ignorant of the treatment given when the decision is made.

Sometimes it is necessary to use a more sophisticated design. Perhaps the two types of tablets differ in appearance or perhaps the dosage or time intervals differ. In that case it is necessary to manufacture dummy tablets looking like drug A and dummy tablets looking like drug B. Then it is possible to preserve blindness by using the so-called double-dummy technique, according to which the patients in one group receive drug A + placebo B and those in the other drug B + placebo A.

The reader of the report should always ask himself whether or not the blinding was successful. Sometimes it is stated that the trial was double-blind when, in fact, in some cases either the patient or the doctor had guessed which treatment was given. One of the drugs may have an acid taste, discolour the urine or be associated with other characteristic effects. In one allegedly double-blind trial of peppermint oil capsules against irritable bowel symptoms, some of the patients reported that members of their family had noticed the smell of peppermint when they had used the w.c. Problems of this kind are particularly likely to occur in cross-over trials (see below) where the patients' experience both treatments, and it is advisable to ask all patients on their last visit what their guess is as regards the treatment they received and what the basis is for their assumption.

The blinding technique may require modification if it is necessary to individualize the number of tablets given to each patient according to the treatment response. Oral anticoagulant treatment, for instance, requires frequent adjustment of the dose, for which reason the standard design cannot be used. Instead the trial is designed in such a way that one doctor, who has no personal contact with the patients, adjusts the dose of anticoagulant tablets in the actively treated patients and, in a similar fashion, alters the dosage of the dummy tablets in the control group. Then a different clinician may record the treatment effect without knowing to which treatment group the patients belong.

A similar situation occurs when surgeons wish to compare two different surgical procedures. Here the surgeons cannot, of course, be blinded, but the problem is solved if somebody else, for instance a physician, assesses the treatment result. Similarly, when the effect of two training programmes for back pain are compared, it is not possible to conceal the nature of the treatment from the patient, but the clinician who assesses the treatment result need not know which treatment was given.

It can sometimes be useful to do trials where only the patients are blinded, if the patients themselves assess their condition. A trial compared laparoscopic cholecystectomy with small-incision cholecystectomy by laparotomy, and the patients and nurses were kept blind as similar bandages were used in all cases. It is commonly believed that laparoscopic surgery, although it takes longer, has the advantage that the patients can be discharged from hospital much earlier, but in this trial where the blinded patients decided for themselves when they felt ready to go home, the length of the hospital stay was the same in the two groups.[150]

It follows from this discussion that often it is not possible to do perfectly blinded trials, and in all such cases the investigators can do no more than choose that technique which reduces the risk of bias as much as at all possible. It is often feasible to blind part of the assessment, e.g. the reading of X-ray films or the physical examination of the patient. The risk of bias depends on the measures of effect and thus it varies from trial to trial. The patients' own assessment of their subjective symptoms is of course much more sensitive to bias than determinations of survival time or other objective observations but, unfortunately, the objective measures of effect may sometimes be less relevant from a clinical point of view than the subjective ones.

Both randomization and blinding are very important tools for the prevention of bias, and of these the former is the more important. Randomization can always be done properly whereas perfect blinding is an ideal that sometimes can be attained, especially in drug trials.

Cross-over trials

The design that has been discussed so far is the group comparative trial, where the patients are allocated to an experimental group or a control group. If, however, the disease is of long duration, and if the treatment only alleviates the symptoms, but does not alter the course of the disease, it may be worthwhile to design a cross-over trial where each patient provides his own control. According to this design all patients are given both treatments, for instance the new and the old drug, in succession, and the response to the two treatments is recorded and compared. This kind of trial also requires randomization, ensuring that the treatment order varies at random, and, if possible, blinding so that patients and clinicians are unaware which treatment is given during which period.

The interval between the administration of the drug and the onset of effect must be short and the effect must subside quickly after cessation of medication, i.e. there must be no carry-over effect to the next treatment period.

It must also be remembered that patients with chronic diseases usually turn to their doctor when their symptoms are at their worst, and therefore it is often seen that the patients' symptoms tend to improve more in one of the periods regardless of the treatment given. This phenomenon is called a period effect. Occasionally the reports of cross-over trials are so detailed that it is possible for the reader to detect carry-over or period effects which were overlooked by the authors.

It is usually stated that cross-over trials require fewer patients than group comparative trials, since the patients serve as their own controls and the between-patient variation has been eliminated. Sometimes, however, the symptoms fluctuate so much that this design provides no advantage over the simpler group comparative design. The interpretation of the results can also be difficult when patients drop out of the trial in the first period and do not try the treatment in the second period, or when a harm develops slowly and is not registered before the second period.

Measures of benefits and harms

The clinical data that serve to measure the treatment effects must be as reliable as possible, as regards both their reproducibility and their accuracy, but, first of all, they must be clinically relevant. This topic, which was discussed in some detail in Chapter 2, is of particular importance for the planning and interpretation of randomized clinical trials.

In many trials the choice of outcome measures is uncontroversial. Antiviral drugs used for the treatment of herpes zoster must be tested for their effects on the pain and the rash, and in trials with antiepileptic drugs one must consider the frequency and severity of epileptic fits. In other studies, however, the situation is rather more complex. In trials of cancer chemotherapy, for instance, it is not sufficient to determine the survival time. One must also record the occurrence and severity of a variety of symptoms, both those caused by the disease and those caused by the treatment, and global assessments of the patients' clinical condition may be appropriate, preferably using simple rating scales.

Clinical research workers often show considerable ingenuity when they choose the outcome measures, and they may go too far. Previously, the most common effect measure in trials of antirheumatic drugs was grip strength.[151] Patients were asked to squeeze the inflated cuff of a sphygmomanometer to permit the measurement of grip strength in mm Hg. Perhaps it is found that one drug causes a greater increase in the grip strength than the other and perhaps this difference is statistically significant, but it is by no means certain that an increase from, say, 120 to 130 mmHg has any clinical significance whatsoever.[151] It might have been better to focus on the patients' ability to cope with their daily chores and such outcomes are now commonly used. Other irrelevant effect measures in arthritis trials were mentioned on p. 15.

Sometimes *surrogate outcome measures* are used, i.e. outcome measures that are not clinically relevant *per se*, but are believed to be good indicators of the clinically relevant outcome, and this may be justified in some cases. For instance, gastroenterologists have tested different drug combinations for the eradication of Helicobacter pylori in patients with duodenal ulcers. Usually, the Helicobacter infection causes no symptoms at all, and the true aim of the treatment is to prevent ulcer recurrence. Therefore, successful eradication is a surrogate outcome, but it is an acceptable one as it has been shown in other studies that ulcer recurrences in Helicobacter-negative people are extremely rare.

The use of surrogate outcomes is often doubtful, however.[149] I have already mentioned (p. 35) the trial of fluoride treatment in cases of osteoporosis where the bone mineral content served as a surrogate outcome in the belief that an increased content would lower the risk of fractures. However, fluoride treatment, which had the desired effect on the surrogate outcome, also led to an increased risk of fractures.

The introduction of new antiarrhythmic drugs in the 1980s is one of the most frightening examples of the dire results of using a surrogate measure. Certain types of ventricular dysrhythmias arising after a myocardial infarction predispose to ventricular fibrillation and death from cardiogenic shock. Therefore, it was taken for granted that the new drugs which, in randomized trials, were found to restore the normal cardiac rhythm in patients with dysrhythmia, would also prevent sudden cardiac deaths, and soon they were widely used after an acute myocardial infarction. However, a number of unexpected deaths raised the suspicion that the drugs were not safe, and finally they were tested in a randomized clinical trial where the outcome was not the immediate antiarrhythmic effect, but the effect on survival. It turned out that in some patients the drugs produced arrythmias and the net result of their use was that the risk of death rose rather than fell.[152] The treatment was used extensively in the United States and it has been estimated that it caused the death of more than 50 000 people per year in that country alone, i.e. more than the American loss of lives during the Vietnam War.[153]

A more recent example of the disasters of relying on surrogate outcomes is the widespread use of hormone replacement therapy. The treatment's name is seductive as it implies that, although being a natural phenomenon, the decrease in hormonal activity at menopause should be viewed as a deficiency that needs replacement, just as patients with diabetes need replacement with insulin. As the hormones have beneficial effects on blood lipids, it was believed that they would prevent cardiac disease, but when large randomized trials were ultimately performed, it was revealed that they increased the incidence of cardiac disease.[154]

These examples illustrate that the interaction between disease mechanisms and the mechanisms of action of different treatments is so complex that it is dangerous not to record directly the clinically relevant outcomes. However, it is easy to understand that clinical research workers often feel tempted to use surrogate measures. The effect of an antihypertensive drug on the blood pressure is seen quickly, and relatively few patients with dysrhythmia are needed to ascertain that a drug has an antiarrhythmic effect. Much longer follow-up periods and many more patients are required to record the clinically relevant effects on prognosis and survival, and, not to forget, to identify the various harms of the treatment. Those who favour surrogate outcomes tend to ignore that all treatments can do harm as they usually design trials that only aim to describe the expected benefits.

Sometimes the distinction between surrogate measures and clinically relevant outcomes is not quite simple. It is, for instance, well established that bronchoconstriction plays a causal role in acute asthma, and therefore it may be reasonable to use the results of spirometry as measures of effect in trials of different bronchodilators. Even in this case, however, many clinicians drew the wrong conclusions. They overlooked that the results did not support the use of long-term treatment. Previously, it was customary to advise asthma patients to use their inhaler four times daily regardless of their clinical condition, but this advice disregarded the fact that the true aim of such treatment is to lower the future risk of admission to hospital with acute asthma attacks and to lower the risk of death. It has now been shown that treatment with long-acting β-agonists increases the number of asthma-related deaths.[155]

Papers reporting randomized trials must also provide information about harms. Patients taking part in trials will be monitored regularly by careful questioning and in drug trials often also by paraclinical tests, e.g. blood and urine analyses aimed at detecting damage to the liver, kidney or bone marrow.

Some participants may complain of mild symptoms, such as headache, dyspepsia, diarrhoea or dizziness, and the frequency of these complaints may well be the same in the treatment group and in a control group where the patients only receive inert tablets. Nevertheless, all subjective symptoms must be recorded, and their severity must be noted.

Careful monitoring is particularly essential when new drugs are being tested, as there is always a risk of serious harms. Unfortunately, however, the reporting of harms is generally insufficient and the preferred terminology underlines just how unwelcome harms are. The effects of drugs are usually described with the terms *efficacy* and *safety*, both of which are positively laden words. We should instead speak of their benefits and harms.[156]

The interest in harms can influence substantially what we find. For instance, more than 10 times as many ulcers were reported in recent trials where selective antirheumatic drugs with fewer gastrointestinal harms were compared with old antirheumatic drugs, than in older trials where old antirheumatic drugs were compared with placebo.[157] However, in the more recent trials the patients underwent regular endoscopy and minor changes that lacked clinical relevance were recorded as 'ulcers'. This doubtful tactic contributed to discrediting the older drugs.

The sample size of a randomized clinical trial must be so large that clinically significant, beneficial effects are not likely to be missed, but it is rarely large enough to detect rare harms. Drug treatment of a trivial disease is, of course, quite unacceptable if one patient in 400 dies of a serious harm, but a simple calculation will show that there is only a 30% probability that this event will occur if the treatment group comprises 500 patients. Therefore, it is very important that medical practitioners watch out for all unexpected events when they start using a new drug and that they report these to the relevant authority.

Stopping rules

It must be decided in advance when a randomized trial is to stop, i.e. when no more patients are to be admitted. The correct procedure is to declare the necessary sample size in the protocol and to stop the trial when that number of patients has been reached. Otherwise, if the trial is not blinded, the investigators may be tempted to look at the results in the two treatment groups from time to time and then stop the trial when they feel convinced that the new treatment is better than the old one. That is of course quite impermissible. If two treatments are equally effective and if the results in the two groups are compared repeatedly throughout the trial, it is only to be expected that the new treatment from time to time, simply by chance, will have provided better results than the old one. To conclude the trial when that has happened is equivalent to the introduction of new rules for the next soccer game between England and Denmark: the game is stopped as soon as Denmark is in the lead, but it continues if the two teams are even, or if England is in the lead. Undoubtedly, the English supporters would object strongly to this idea. Unfortunately, those clinical research workers who use that kind of stopping rule are unlikely to write it in their paper, and the reader of the article will be misled.

But there is no rule without exceptions. It may be desirable for ethical reasons to ensure that the trial can be stopped prematurely, if the difference between the treatment results in the two groups proves to be particularly large or if one of the treatments causes serious harms. That possibility must, however, be foreseen at the planning stage by the establishment of an independent safety monitoring committee, i.e. a committee of experts not associated with the running of the trial, who may look at the results at regular intervals. It must be stated in the protocol which statistical calculations they should do (usually a so-called group sequential analysis) and at what times, and under which circumstances they are authorized to stop the trial.

Unfortunately, most trials that are stopped early do not live up to these standards at all, and the reader therefore needs to view the results of such trials with scepticism.[158]

Assessment of the results

The assessment of the results after the completion of the trial invariably involves subjective judgments. Researchers therefore need to report in detail what they did.[143,156,159,160] Inspection of the information about each individual patient will probably reveal that some of them did not fulfil the requirements of the protocol, as some may have missed one or more of the stipulated visits to the clinic, while others did not take the drug as prescribed. Those patients who did not complete the trial as planned or did not take the tablets at all are recorded as *drop-outs*, but in less clear cases it is a matter of choice whether or not the patients should be labelled as such. Therefore, in order to prevent bias, those who make the decisions about what to do with the often less-than-perfect data ought not know to which treatment group the patients belong, but unfortunately this rule has not yet gained general acceptance. A survey of randomized trials of antirheumatic drugs revealed many examples of bias in connection with the analysis and the interpretation of the results that, almost without exception, favoured the new drug over the active control drug.[29]

The inspection of the database and the sorting out of the ambiguities serve the purpose of producing a so-called 'clean data file' that can be subjected to numerical analysis of the results. The handling of the drop-outs and other problems with missing data may, however, cause serious problems. The simplest solution is to do a *per protocol analysis* which only includes those patients who completed the trial as planned, but the exclusion of the drop-outs will usually introduce bias. Perhaps some of those patients who received the new treatment did not turn up for the scheduled visits because the treatment did not help them at all or perhaps they felt so well that the visits did not seem worthwhile. Mostly, however, patients who dropped out fared worse than other patients, and therefore a per protocol analysis will generally tend to overestimate the effect.[161]

The *intention-to-treat analysis* is much more reliable and it also reflects what happens in practice, namely that some patients will not take all of the prescribed treatment. Here, all patients who entered the two treatment groups are included, whether or not they completed the trial according to the protocol. This type of analysis is realistic, if it is possible to record the outcome in all patients, including the drop-outs. That was the case in a large trial of acetylsalicylic acid, given to patients with atrial fibrillation in order to prevent major cerebrovascular accidents, where all cases of stroke, including those among the drop-outs, could be retrieved by means of various registers. In some trials, however, this is not possible. Some years ago numerous trials were done, which compared the effect of different H_2-blockers and proton pump inhibitors on the healing of peptic ulcers, and one could not possibly know whether or not the ulcer had healed if the patient did not turn up for the gastroscopy at the end of treatment. Usually, it was assumed in the intention-to-treat analyses that the ulcer had remained unhealed in all drop-outs, and obviously that assumption was unwarranted. In order to be on the safe side, the clinician might have made the rather unreasonable assumption that the ulcers of the drop-outs in the treatment group had remained unhealed whereas those in the control group had healed.

One should always perform one or more intention-to-treat analyses, making different assumptions. These analyses may be supplemented with a per protocol analysis, but it is not strictly necessary, and one should bear in mind that such an analysis can be quite misleading.

Different authors may define intention-to-treat quite differently,[162] and, particularly in industry-sponsored drug trials, a number of patients have often been omitted from the analyses, in which case this term should not be used.

Statistical analysis

Hypothesis testing

It is not sufficient to quote the average results in each treatment group. The results must be subjected to a statistical analysis in order to assess the possible influence of random variation, and the principle is best explained by means of a numerical example.

Table 6.1a shows the results of a group comparative trial with 300 patients in each treatment group. Two hundred and forty, or 80%, of those patients who received drug A were cured compared with 210, or 70%, of those who

Table 6.1 Results of three randomised trials.

a)

	Cured	Not cured	Total
Treatment A	240	60	300
Treatment B	210	90	300
Total	450	150	600

b)

	Cured	Not cured	Total
Treatment A	233	67	300
Treatment B	210	90	300
Total	443	157	600

c)

	Cured	Not cured	Total
Treatment A	226	74	300
Treatment B	210	90	300
Total	436	164	600

were treated with drug B. Consequently, the difference between the cure rates
is 10%. These results suggest that treatment A is more efficient than treatment
B, but we cannot exclude the possibility that they are in fact equally effective
and that the difference arose by chance. The third possibility, that treatment B
is better than treatment A, is also possible, but it is far less likely and will not
be considered below.

The statistical analysis of the results of the trial begins with the formulation
of two hypotheses, which are denoted the *null hypothesis* and the *alternative
hypothesis*. According to the null hypothesis, the two treatments are equally
good (the observed difference between the results is due to random variation)
and, according to the alternative hypothesis, treatment A and treatment B have
different effects. The clinician who has to make the choice between treatment A
and treatment B cannot know which of the two hypotheses is true, but in spite
of that he has to make up his mind which treatment he is going to prescribe
in the future. The situation is illustrated by Table 6.2, in which H_0 denotes the
null hypothesis and H_A the alternative hypothesis. It is seen that there are four
possibilities depending on the truth and the clinician's choice:

1. The physician decides to act as if the two treatments are equally good, and
   the two treatments *are* equally good. He accepts a true null hypothesis and
   commits no error.
2. The physician decides to act as if treatment A is better than treatment B, but
   the truth is that the two treatments are equally good. He rejects a true null
   hypothesis, and consequently he makes a mistake. In statistical terminology
   this mistake is called a type I error (an error of the first kind, or an α-error).
3. The physician decides to act as if the two treatments are equally good, but
   the truth is that treatment A is better than treatment B. He accepts a false
   null hypothesis, and in statistical terms he is committing a type II error (an
   error of the second kind, or a β-error).

Table 6.2 Type I and type II errors.

		Truth	
		$H_A: A \neq B$	$H_0: A = B$
Physician's choice	$H_A: A \neq B$	No error	Type I error
	$H_0: A = B$	Type II error	No error

4. The physician decides to act as if treatment A is better than treatment B, and treatment A *is* better than treatment B. He rejects a false null hypothesis and commits no error.

The distinction between type I and type II errors is important, but admittedly it is rather difficult to remember which is which. Perhaps the following mnemonic will be of some help. A doctor studies the results of a randomized trial and wonders whether or not he should reject the null hypothesis that the new treatment is no better than the old one. If he is an optimist he will be easily convinced, and if the null hypothesis is true he will have committed a type I error. If, however, he is a pessimist he may be more difficult to convince and he may stick to the null hypothesis in spite of the fact that the new drug is better. Then he is committing a type II error. O precedes P as I precedes II, and therefore the 'optimist error' is a type I error and the 'pessimist error' is a type II error.

It now remains to consider to what extent the actual results of the trial are compatible with the two hypotheses, H_0 and H_A, and for this purpose it is customary to do a suitable *significance test*. Here I shall not discuss the mathematics of the tests, but the procedure is as follows: we make the assumption that the two treatments are identical, i.e. that the null hypothesis is true, and then we calculate the probability of obtaining, by chance, a difference between the treatment results which, numerically, is as large as or larger than the one observed in the trial. The choice of the statistical test depends on the problem at hand (see Chapter 8), and in this case it would be appropriate to use Fisher's exact test (or a χ^2-test). We shall find that P = 0.006, and this result must be interpreted as follows:

The probability (P) of obtaining a difference between the cure rates of 10% or more, either in favour of treatment A or in favour of treatment B, if the null hypothesis were true, is 0.006.

If treatment A had cured seven less patients (Table 6.1b) the difference between the two cure rates would only have been 8%, and the statistical analysis would have shown that P = 0.04, i.e. that the chance of obtaining at least such a difference, if the null hypothesis were true, would be 4%. In the third example (Table 6.1c), the number of patients cured by treatment A has once again been reduced by seven, and now the difference between the cure rates is only 5%. The P-value would be 0.17, i.e. there would be a 17% probability of obtaining at least such a difference, if the treatments were in fact equally effective. Under those circumstances the clinician might decide to act as if the null hypothesis were true, and by doing so he would either be right or he would be committing a type II error.

According to convention, a difference is said to be *statistically significant*, if the P-value is less than 5%. Therefore, we may say that treatment A gave significantly better results than treatment B in the first two examples, but not in the third, and it is often implied by these expressions that in the first two examples the clinician ought to accept that the new treatment is more effective, whereas in the third he ought to accept the null hypothesis. Sometimes it is almost regarded as 'unscientific' to believe in a result that is statistically non-significant, or not to believe in one that is statistically significant. This convention, however, is most unfortunate, as it may well lead to a mental block that prevents the correct interpretation of the calculated P-values. This important point is best explained by an example.

Imagine that we hear about a trial which compares the effect of tablets made from a particular herb and inert tablets on the survival time of patients suffering from a particular kind of cancer. We are well acquainted with the literature on the topic and the available scientific evidence makes us conclude that there is only one chance in a thousand that the herb is effective. In other words, we attribute the alternative hypothesis a probability of 0.1%. Then imagine that the trial is completed and that the results are those shown in Table 6.1b. The difference is statistically significant as the P-value is slightly less than 5%, but irrespective of that result we should not suddenly change our minds and conclude that the herb is effective. Our prior confidence in the alternative hypothesis was only 0.1%, and we should not be convinced by a result that is likely to occur in almost 5% of trials when the null hypothesis is true.

This problem is analogous to the one that was discussed on p. 101 in connection with the interpretation of confidence intervals and it shows that we must distinguish between frequential (statistical) probabilities and subjective probabilities. The statistician asks the following question: 'What is the frequential probability of obtaining the observed results (or even more extreme results), if the null hypothesis is true?', and the P-value is the answer.

The reader of the medical journal who has to make up his mind whether or not to believe in the efficacy of the drug asks the reverse question: What is the probability that the null hypothesis is true, now that I have seen the reported results? This is a subjective probability and it depends not only on the P-value, but also on one's prior confidence in the null hypothesis and the alternative hypothesis.

Attempts have been made to formalize this type of reasoning by means of Bayesian statistics, but here we shall only suggest a simple rule-of-thumb: One should not reject the null hypothesis, if the P-value is larger than our prior confidence in the alternative hypothesis.

However, the decision not to be persuaded by the result does not necessarily imply that it should be ignored. If, later, we read about other studies that have a similar outcome, we shall remember the results in the first report and be less sceptical towards the treatment.

Similar reasoning is appropriate if the statistical analysis resulted in a non-significant P-value and if our prior confidence in the alternative hypothesis was high. This might be the case if a new drug had already been shown to possess the same biological properties as other similar drugs, which are effective. If the number of patients is small, we may decide, in spite of a large P-value, that probably the treatment is effective and that we should commit a type II error if we concluded otherwise. In Chapter 8 (p. 199) these arguments will be illustrated by a numerical example.

P-values are frequently misinterpreted, and some doctors even mistake statistical significance for clinical significance. They believe that a small P-value is equivalent to a large clinical effect. That is, of course, a misunderstanding. If Table 6.1a showed the effect of two treatments on the survival of patients with a malignant disease, we should say that the difference was highly significant from a clinical point of view, whereas we should be less impressed if it showed the difference between the antipruritic effects of two ointments for haemorrhoids. The importance of a given difference depends on the clinical problem. It should also be born in mind that a difference between the treatment effects in two groups will become statistically significant, no matter how small it is, if only the number of patients is sufficiently large.

Estimation

Conventional significance tests have the limitation that they only help the clinician to decide whether or not the effect of a new treatment differs from that of an old one. They do not answer the question: How much better (or how much worse) is the new treatment? In order to extract that information from the results of a randomized trial, we shall have to estimate the therapeutic gain or, in other words, we must calculate the 95% confidence interval of the observed difference.[163] With a term borrowed from risk factor epidemiology, this is usually called the *risk difference*. However, as the outcomes are often desired ones, e.g. survival or cure, it seems somewhat awkward to describe them as risks.

Consider once again the first of the three numerical examples (Table 6.1a) where the observed difference between the treatment effects, i.e. the observed therapeutic gain, was 10%. The calculation of the 95% confidence interval of an observed rate was mentioned on p. 101, and the 95% confidence interval of the difference between two rates can be calculated in much the same way. In this case it will be found that the 95% confidence interval is 3% to 17%, which suggests that the therapeutic gain is at least 3% and at most 17%. However, the calculated confidence interval only includes the true therapeutic gain in 19 out of 20 trials, and, when judging the results of a particular trial, we should always consider the possibility that we are faced with the 'twentieth trial' where the true therapeutic gain is lower than the lower confidence limit or higher than the higher limit. The results of other studies or other kinds of information may suggest that this is the case.

In the example in Table 6.1b the observed therapeutic gain had been reduced to 8%, and a calculation will show that now the 95% confidence interval is 1% to 15%. Therefore, according to this calculation, the therapeutic gain is at least 1% and at most 15%. In Table 6.1c the therapeutic gain is even smaller, i.e. 5%, and the 95% confidence interval is −2% to 12%. This means that by using treatment A instead of treatment B one may expect to cure between 2% fewer patients and 12% more patients.

The confidence intervals agree well with the P-values, which is only to be expected as the calculations are based on similar principles. In the first two examples the interval did not include zero, and the P-value was statistically significant ($P < 0.05$); both results suggest that the null hypothesis should be rejected. In the third example the interval included zero and the P-value was statistically non-significant, suggesting that the null hypothesis should not be rejected.

The calculated confidence intervals of the therapeutic gain are especially revealing if the number of patients is small. Imagine a randomized trial of 60 patients where 15 of 30 patients who received treatment A were cured compared with 12 of 30 patients who received treatment B. The therapeutic gain is 10%, just as in Table 6.1a, but now the 95% confidence interval is −15% to 35%. According to this calculation treatment A may cure up to 35% more patients than treatment B, but it is not excluded that it cures 15% fewer patients. A significance test would only show that the null hypothesis might well be true, but it provides no information as regards the possible size of the difference.

Today all leading medical journals require that the authors quote the confidence intervals.[164] This can easily be done (with some approximation) using the following formula:

$$TG \pm 2\sqrt{\frac{p_1(1-p_1)}{N_1} + \frac{p_2(1-p_2)}{N_2}}$$

Where p_1 and p_2 are the cure rates and N_1 and N_2 the number of patients in each group. TG is the therapeutic gain ($p_1 - p_2$).

Other statistical measures of effect

The therapeutic gain, i.e. the difference between the two cure rates, is the most relevant statistical measure of effect from a clinical point of view, but there are also other possibilities.

When, as in this case, we are dealing with data on a binary scale (cured/not cured) one may also calculate the *relative risk (RR)*. This statistical measure is used, for instance, in randomized clinical trials of treatments that serve to prevent death where it seems more natural to talk about the 'risk of death' than the 'cure rate'. The RR is also calculated in other types of randomized trials, however. If, once again, we look at the figures in Table 6.1a it will be noted that the risk of *not* being cured was 20% in treatment group A and 30% in group B, and consequently the relative risk in favour of treatment A was 0.20/0.30 = 0.67. One may also calculate the confidence interval or do a significance test in order to assess whether the observed relative risk differs significantly from one.

In spite of its popularity this statistical measure is unsatisfactory from a clinical point of view. A relative risk of 0.67 does not tell us whether the risk of not being cured (as in this case) was reduced from 30% to 20% or whether it was reduced from, say, 0.3% to 0.2%, which is the most optimistic effect estimate that has been reported after 10 years of screening for breast cancer with mammography.[53] In order to remedy this deficiency, it has been suggested that one should also calculate the *number needed to treat* (or *NNT*),[16] i.e. the number of patients who must be treated in order to cure (or extend the life of) one patient. This number is simply the reciprocal of the therapeutic gain (or risk difference). Thus, NNT = 1/0.1 = 10, if the risk is reduced from 30% to 20%, and NNT = 1/0.001 = 1000, if the risk is reduced from 0.3% to 0.2%. The number needed to treat may also be calculated directly from the figures in the fourfold table. Table 6.1a shows that 30 more patients were cured in group A than in group B. The number of patients in each group was 300, which means that it was necessary to treat 300/30 = 10 patients with treatment A in order to obtain one additional cure.

Effects measured on an ordinal or an interval scale require other statistical methods (see Chapter 8). Life table statistics are used to assess the survival time using different treatments (see Chapter 8).

Subgroup analyses

When a randomized clinical trial has been completed, it is tempting to 'go fishing'. The total sample of patients is divided up into subgroups and the effect of the two treatments is compared for women alone, for men, for patients with particular symptoms, for old people etc. That, of course, is a doubtful undertaking as, predictably, one in 20 of such subgroup comparisons will turn out to be statistically significant simply by chance, even when the null hypothesis is true. Further, subgroup analyses do not only invite type I errors, but also type II errors. If the trial as a whole revealed a significant difference between the treatment results, it cannot be expected that this difference will repeat itself in all subgroups as they have more limited sample sizes.

Nevertheless, papers in medical journals frequently report the results of such 'fishing expeditions', which may well influence the clinical recommendations which are derived from the study. One large trial of the effect of streptokinase in acute myocardial infarction revealed a reduction of the death rate by 20%, but unfortunately the authors did a subgroup analysis and concluded that the treatment was only effective if it was started within six hours of the onset of symptoms, and if the patient was younger than 65 years old and had an anterior infarction.[165] As usual, the conclusions derived from the fishing expedition were later disproved. The authors of a similar mega-trial were so annoyed by such conclusions that they added the result of an astrological subgroup analysis. They noted a decrease in the death rate in the trial as a whole, but added that the treatment was harmful to patients born under the sign of Gemini or Libra.[166]

Systematic reviews

The individual physician seeks to keep his knowledge up-to-date by reading medical journals. It is exciting to read that some new treatment is more effective than the one in current use, and, if the trial is sufficiently large and methodologically acceptable, it may seem justified to adopt the new treatment immediately. Usually, however, a certain amount of healthy scepticism is in its place. Perhaps the trial has major flaws that will be revealed in subsequent letters to the editor, or perhaps the trial was too small to detect rare but serious harms.

There could also be other trials, unknown to the reader, with less encouraging results. Therefore, it is important to read good review articles written by experts who have done a thorough study of the literature in a particular field, but even that kind of information is not always trustworthy. It has been shown repeatedly that some reviews, even in the best medical journals, are biased, as the authors tend to quote only those trials which support their own point of view.[86] It is also common that reviews that appear to have been written by clinical experts, in reality have been written by *ghost authors*, i.e. authors who, although they wrote the paper, do not appear as authors.[167,168] Ghost authors paid by the drug industry are also frequently involved when results from randomized trials are written up.[167–169] It is therefore not surprising that many reviews, editorials and clinical trial reports contain exaggerated claims about the alleged advantages of new drugs.

An additional problem is *publication bias*, which is the phenomenon that trials with a statistically significant result are more likely to be published than those with a non-significant result.[170] Usually, the results of large trials of a high methodological standard will reach the medical journals, regardless of the outcome, but smaller trials, especially those that did not find that the new treatment was better than the old one, may not do so. If the outcome seems uninteresting, the investigators may not feel that it is worthwhile making the effort to analyse their data and to write a paper. It is also common that research findings remain unpublished for commercial reasons.

Systematic reviews are far more reliable than ordinary reviews. Each systematic review aims at creating a comprehensive and unbiased picture of the results of all those randomized clinical trials that address a particular clinical problem. It is a research project in its own right and, like other projects, it requires meticulous planning and a detailed protocol. This protocol describes the entry criteria for those trials that can be included in the review.

In 1993 The Cochrane Collaboration was established by Iain Chalmers in order to promote the production of systematic reviews which are published electronically in The Cochrane Library.[141] The initiative was British, but there are now 12 Cochrane Centres in different parts of the world and 51 international, multi-disciplinary editorial groups that co-ordinate hand-searching of medical journals and abstracts from scientific congresses in order to identify as many trials as possible. Anybody who wishes to contribute can join the collaboration, which is registered as a charity, but those who accept to do systematic reviews are expected to update these on a regular basis.

The database currently contains more than 3000 systematic reviews, as well as more than 400 000 references to controlled trials, and about 15 000 researchers and others from all over the world contribute to the work. Therefore, the database should be consulted by any clinician who in his daily work wishes to assess the available knowledge about a particular intervention.

This massive undertaking builds to a large extent on voluntary, unpaid work, and it owes much of its success to a project in the 1980s that similarly collected and reviewed clinical trials in pregnancy and childbirth.[171]

The search of the literature is crucial as an attempt must be made to find all relevant studies, and the methods used must be described in detail in the review. Then the reader may judge for himself whether or not it was sufficiently thorough. One should not limit the searches to certain languages, but should get articles translated if necessary. Usually an iterative search strategy is developed, where some of the words from the titles and abstracts of the first papers to be retrieved are used for a renewed search. The Cochrane Library should be searched, in addition to other databases such as PubMed, and it is also necessary to use other sources of information. Reference lists of relevant articles should be searched, and it can be useful to write to active researchers in the field and to pharmaceutical companies, although the drug industry is not always very cooperative.

When the different trials are reasonably comparable and their results are not too different, it is often possible to perform a *meta-analysis*[172,173] in which the results from the individual trials are combined to yield an overall estimate of the effect of the treatment. Of course, a meta-analysis should not be done without a prior protocol and a thorough systematic review of the literature. The research literature is riddled with bias that tends to exaggerate the advantages of new interventions, and it is easy to simply reproduce the errors if one is not very careful and has already tried to envisage the potential problems when writing the protocol.[172]

Even with great care there are limitations, as trial authors tend to publish outcome measures selectively. Comparisons of trial protocols with published articles have shown that there are often more outcomes than those reported, and that outcomes are more often published fully when they are statistically significant.[174] This, of course, introduces a bias that the meta-analyst cannot compensate for. Meta-analyses are therefore generally too positive and outcome reporting bias can only be avoided if it becomes mandatory that all results from all trials be publicly available.

Fig. 6.1 illustrates graphically the result of a Cochrane review based on 14 randomized clinical trials comparing somatostatin and similar drugs with placebo or no treatment in patients with bleeding oesophageal varices.[112] The table shows for each trial the total number of patients (N) and the number of patients who died (n) in the treatment group and in the control group. The relative risk (RR) of dying, with the 95% confidence interval, is also shown for each trial, both numerically and graphically. The width of the confidence interval reflects the number of deaths (many deaths give narrow intervals). For

Review: Somatostatin analogues for acute bleeding oesophageal varices
Comparison: 01 Somatostatin analogues versus placebo or no treatment
Outcome: 01 Mortality

Study	Treatment n/N	Control n/N	Relative Risk (Fixed) 95% CI	Weight (%)	Relative Risk (Fixed) 95% CI
01 Randomisation concealed, double-blind trials					
Avgerinos 1997	27/101	24/104		12.0	1.16 [0.72, 1.87]
Besson 1995	12/98	12/101		6.0	1.03 [0.49, 2.18]
Burroughs 1990	9/61	7/59		3.6	1.24 [0.50, 3.12]
Calés 2001	17/109	25/115		12.4	0.72 [0.41, 1.25]
Gotzsche 1995	16/42	16/44		7.9	1.05 [0.61, 1.81]
Moretó 1994	3/33	6/30		3.2	0.45 [0.12, 1.66]
Zuberi 2000	1/35	1/35		0.5	1.00 [0.07, 15.36]
Subtotal (95% CI)	479	488		45.6	0.96 [0.74, 1.24]
Total events: 85 (Treatment), 91 (Control)					
Test for heterogeneity chi-square=3.36 df=6 p=0.76 I²=0.0%					
Test for overall effect z=0.32 p=0.8					
02 Other trials					
Burroughs 1996	42/189	53/194		26.6	0.81 [0.57, 1.16]
Farooqi 2000	1/69	6/72		3.0	0.17 [0.02, 1.41]
Pauwels 1994	7/18	5/14		2.9	1.09 [0.44, 2.71]
Shiha 1996	7/93	8/96		4.0	0.90 [0.34, 2.39]
Souza 2003	10/56	13/56		6.6	0.77 [0.37, 1.61]
Sung 1995	5/47	11/47		5.6	0.45 [0.17, 1.21]
Valenzuela 1989	15/48	10/36		5.8	1.13 [0.57, 2.21]
Subtotal (95% CI)	520	515		54.4	0.79 [0.61, 1.02]
Total events: 87 (Treatment), 106 (Control)					
Test for heterogeneity chi-square=4.88 df=6 p=0.56 I²=0.0%					
Test for overall effect z=1.83 p=0.07					
Total (95% CI)	999	1003		100.0	0.87 [0.72, 1.04]
Total events: 172 (Treatment), 197 (Control)					
Test for heterogeneity chi-square=9.07 df=13 p=0.77 I²=0.0%					
Test for overall effect z=1.54 p=0.1					

0.1 0.2 0.5 1 2 5 10

Favours drug   Favours control

Fig. 6.1 The result of a meta-analysis of 14 randomized trials comparing somatostatin and similar drugs with placebo or no treatment in patients with bleeding oesophageal varices. As shown with the diamonds, there was no statistically significant reduction in mortality (4% in the best trials, 95% confidence interval 26% reduction to 24% increase). The most important statistical calculations are explained in the text.

all the trials taken together, this interval comprised one, which means that the result was not statistically significant.

It can be seen that the trials were divided in two groups. In the upper part, the allocation of the patients was concealed and the treatment was labelled double-blind by the trial authors; in the lower part, the trials were of less satisfactory quality. An overall estimate for all the trials was obtained by a statistical procedure that weighs those trials with most deaths the highest. With this analysis, the seven best trials showed a relative risk of 0.96 and a P-value of 0.75. The confidence interval was quite wide and it is possible that a 26% reduction is mortality, or a 24% increase, was overlooked. The analysis of the seven methodologically weaker trials showed a more positive effect with a relative risk of 0.79 and a smaller P-value of only 0.07. The estimate for all 14 trials is shown at the bottom of the figure. It contains no important additional information and one should always rely most on the best trials.

Before the meta-analysis was performed, it was judged whether the variation in the results was too large to justify a meta-analysis. For this purpose, a heterogeneity test was used, and this was non-significant in both groups of trials and for the combined analysis of all 14 trials. However, such a test has very low power when there are few trials, and one should therefore not use the test alone to judge the feasibility of a meta-analysis.

Instead of the relative risk, the authors could also have calculated the therapeutic gain, and in some cases authors show the odds ratio although it is more difficult to interpret (see Chapter 8).

If the number of trials is sufficiently large, it is useful to look at the distribution of the results in a graph where the effect is shown on the x-axis and the precision (corresponding to the number of deaths) on the y-axis. Because of the randomization procedure, it is only to be expected that the results of smaller trials will show greater variation than those of larger trials, but the distribution of the results will be symmetrical if the variation is purely random (Fig. 6.2a).[151,175] If, however, the distribution is asymmetrical, the sample of trials included in the meta-analysis is biased. When this is the case, the most common reason is that the small trials show larger effects than the big trials, as in Fig. 6.2b. Such skewness suggests publication bias, i.e. the fact that some small trials with unfavourable results never reached the medical journals. The example illustrates that one needs to interpret a meta-analysis cautiously if it is only based on small trials. When only small trials were available, a meta-analysis was published that concluded that magnesium was very effective in the treatment of myocardial infarction, but this treatment was later abandoned.

One should, of course, not pool the data in a meta-analysis if the results from the individual trials are very different or if the distribution is asymmetric,

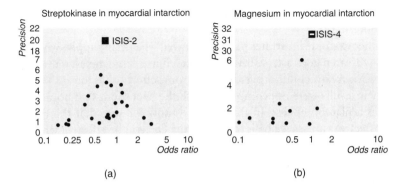

Fig. 6.2 a) Effect of streptokinase in myocardial infarction compared with no treatment, the figure is symmetrical. b) Effect of magnesium in myocardial infarction compared with no treatment, the figure is strongly asymmetrical. The precision increases with the number of deaths and an odds ratio below one means fewer deaths in the treatment group (From *BMJ* 1997;**315**:629–34, reproduced with permission).

as in Fig. 6.2b. However, what is most important is not the statistical analysis, but the fact that the literature was reviewed systematically, based on a detailed protocol. Even without any calculations such a systematic review will be much more reliable than ordinary review articles.

Systematic reviews present other difficulties that must be foreseen and addressed in the protocol. Methodologically flawed trials must be excluded, the criteria for the assessment of their potential for bias having been specified in advance, and it must be decided whether the trials are sufficiently comparable to include them in the same statistical analysis. Otherwise the sample of trials must be subdivided into subgroups.

A systematic review is an efficient tool for assessing the aggregate knowledge of the benefits and harms of a particular treatment at a given moment, but it is, of course, not infallible. There may be hidden sources of bias in the individual trials that cannot be detected even by careful reading of the report, and publication bias and selective reporting of outcomes can never be fully excluded. Subjective judgments are inevitable and it is therefore not surprising that two systematic reviews of the same treatment have sometimes yielded different results, but usually it will be found that one of them was methodologically deficient in one way or another, or that some of the authors had a conflict of interest. For instance, a meta-analysis that was supported by the manufacturer of an antirheumatic drug, rofecoxib, showed that it did not increase the risk of arterial thrombosis,[176] even though the available trials in fact showed the opposite.[145]

The company withdrew the drug from the market three years later because of this serious harm.

Another example illustrates particularly well what may happen when meta-analytic research goes astray. It was concluded in a large meta-analysis of homoeopathic treatment that, overall, it had some effect (or as the authors put it: That their results were not compatible with the hypothesis that homoeopathy only has a placebo effect). In this case we know for sure that the treatment was ineffective (unless we believe that a drug can still be effective when it has been removed by repeated dilution) and therefore this study reveals the combined effect of different sources of bias both in the individual trials and in the combined analysis.[139] The meta-analysts faced the problem of publication bias (which they tried to tackle statistically), but they included studies of a large variety of very different clinical problems, and they admitted that two-thirds of the included trials were methodologically poor. Like others, they found that the higher the quality, the smaller the effect.[177,178]

In retrospect, there can be no doubt that meta-analyses could have saved many lives, if they had been done at the proper time. Streptokinase for acute myocardial infarction, for instance, could have been introduced 10–15 years earlier, if the community of cardiologists had been able to take a comprehensive view of the available evidence.[179] In other cases ineffective or harmful treatments could have been abandoned if meta-analytic evidence had been available.

Meta-analyses also play an important role in clinical research. There are many examples of trials being repeated again and again in spite of the fact that the problem has already found its solution. This is particularly unacceptable when the many control groups have received placebos.[180,181] Some of these unnecessary trials may have been done for commercial purposes, but sometimes the clinical investigators were simply unaware of the previous studies. At other times the omissions seem more deliberate, as when different groups of investigators repeatedly have not only failed to cite a large number of previous trials, but even the largest trial ever performed.[181] Therefore, it ought to be an indispensable requirement that the protocol for a randomized trial refers to a systematic review of those trials that have already been done.

From trials to practice

The decisions taken in everyday clinical work must, to the greatest possible extent, be based on the results of clinical research. Ideally, no treatment should be prescribed unless it has been demonstrated by randomized clinical trials, and preferably by meta-analyses, that it has the desired effects.

Admittedly, there are exceptions to this rule, as sometimes the effect is so obvious that it would be unreasonable to doubt uncontrolled experience. That was the case when ingestion of raw liver was introduced for the treatment of pernicious anaemia; previously all patients died, and now a complete cure was achieved. Those physicians who first used penicillin in acute streptococcal and pneumococcal infections were also quickly convinced of the efficiency of the new treatment. These are but a few accounts of unquestionable therapeutic breakthroughs, and, undoubtedly, there are more to come. If, for instance, some day in the future, we see the first cures for AIDS or for gastric cancer with liver metastases, we shall be convinced of the efficiency of the new treatment even without the evidence from randomized trials.

Such examples, however, are the exceptions rather than the rule. The breakthroughs are few and far between, and in the vast majority of cases progress in therapy means the introduction of new treatments that are only a little better than those in current use, and under these circumstances the evidence from randomized trials is indispensable. We usually have great hopes when we decide to test a new treatment by doing a randomized trial, but experience shows that, on average, the new treatments that are tested are no better, or only marginally better, than the ones with which they are compared.[151,182–185] Therefore, the need for randomized trials cannot be questioned, but it must be realized that the concept of fully evidence-based clinical practice remains an ideal that can never be attained. Firstly, some diseases or conditions are so rare that it can be very difficult, even in multicentre trials, to collect a sufficient number of patients. Secondly, the treatment response may depend on the stage and manifestations of the disease, and concomitant diseases and treatments, and it is impossible to test all new treatments in every subgroup of patients presenting a particular clinical picture. Thirdly, there are situations where randomization may not be acceptable.

It is can also difficult to do therapeutic trials in malignant diseases. Some patients may not accept the risk of being allocated to an untreated control group, as they cling to the hope that the new treatment is effective and are willing to run the risk of unknown harms. This is a serious dilemma as, on one hand, it requires little empathy to understand this attitude, and, on the other, we must guard future patients against the introduction of new treatments that are ineffective or harmful. When some other treatment is available, it is easier to explain to the patients that it is necessary to do a comparative trial, testing the new treatment against the old one.

However, in spite of these difficulties we could get much closer to the ideal of evidence-based clinical practice than we are today. Most randomized trials are concerned with drug therapy, but new methods of physiotherapy and recommendations about changes in lifestyle should also be tested rigorously. Some new surgical techniques have been subjected to randomized trials, but that is the exception and not the rule. Laparoscopic surgery is just one example of a therapeutic method which has become very popular in spite of the fact that for some conditions there was no good evidence of its superiority, and in Denmark the untimely introduction of a new type of cement (Boneloc) to be used in connection with hip replacements developed into a public scandal. This new product seemed very promising and very quickly it was accepted at departments of orthopaedic surgery both at home and abroad, until it was noted that in many cases the cement started to crumble a few years later. Probably, this complication could not have been predicted, but the number of patients who had to undergo a second operation would have been very much smaller if the use of the cement from the start had been confined to a properly conducted randomized trial.

We could also do better in the case of drug trials. In many countries it is impossible to register a new drug if it has not been tested by means of randomized clinical trials, and the standard of clinical research has improved over the years, but readers of medical journals still frequently come across reports of trials which are much too small to provide reliable results or which are methodologically flawed in one way or another. In addition, there is a great need for many more systematic reviews.

It is also necessary to point out that contemporary clinical research, to an increasing extent, is biased by commercial interests. Clinical research ought to be inspired by those problems that clinicians encounter in their daily work, i.e. by those situations where they have to make a decision in spite of the fact that they do not really know what is best for the patient. Such situations occur frequently: Is thrombolytic treatment warranted in this case of thrombophlebitis and pulmonary embolism, or is treatment with heparin and oral anticoagulants better? And is it advisable to start life-long anticoagulant therapy if the thrombophlebitis recurs? Is it necessary to give this patient penicillin intravenously? We have a shortage of staff, and could we not just as well use penicillin tablets? What is the best treatment of 'restless legs'? Does quinine have any effect at all? Searches in The Cochrane Library will show that some randomized trials have been done addressing these and similar questions, but they are very few and far between compared with the number of trials testing different antirheumatic drugs, different H_2-antagonists and proton pump inhibitors against peptic ulcers, and β-blockers in a variety of diseases. The reason is, of course, that peroral anticoagulants, penicillin tablets and quinine have little commercial interest while the introduction of, for instance, a new antirheumatic drug may yield great profits. Such considerations ought to be quite irrelevant in public health services like those in the UK and the Nordic countries, but today economic constraints and increased bureaucracy make it impossible to do large randomized trials without financial support from external sources.

It is also a problem that some patients refuse to take part in randomized trials. Participation in a trial involves a certain degree of altruism, as the patients are well aware that they themselves may not benefit from the results. This reluctance may reflect the rise of individualism in modern society, but commercialization also plays a role. Altruistic feelings will not induce patients to participate if they feel that the trial is motivated by commercial interests rather than the needs of future patients.

Clinical research workers may counteract this development by regarding their patients, not as objects of research, but as partners in the project. All patients who take part in a randomized trial ought to receive a letter after the conclusion of the project telling them what the trial showed and which treatment they received. That is rarely done.

Evidence-based medicine and commercial pressures

This presentation might evoke the picture of the clinician sitting in front of his computer, entering the patient's clinical data, and then reading on the screen which treatment to give. It would, of course, be very helpful for the continued education of all medical practitioners, if it became possible to link diagnoses, treatments and the results of systematic reviews in the databases, but there would still be a need for individualized clinical judgment. There will always be those cases where the diagnosis is not quite certain, those where the clinical picture is atypical and those where the patient suffers from two or more diseases and where the usual treatments for each of these cannot be combined.

As pointed out in connection with the diagnostic decision process (p. 85), it is no simple matter to use the experience gained from groups of patients for making decisions in an individual case. Clinical trials provide information about the statistical probability, i.e. the frequency of cure in a predefined population, whereas the clinician wishes to assess the subjective probability of cure in an individual patient. A randomized clinical trial may have shown that one treatment cured 20% more patients than another treatment, but this result only indicates that on average the chance of cure was 20% higher in one treatment group than in the other. Usually, the clinician acts on the assumption that his patient will respond as the average patient, but sometimes that is not reasonable. The comparison of a medical and a surgical treatment may have shown that surgery gave the best results, but the clinician who is faced with an elderly, frail patient may well judge that medical treatment will give his patient the best chances. The patient's own wishes may also influence the decision. Some people are frightened by the very idea of a surgical operation and then it might also be advisable to prefer medical treatment. This example shows why evidence-based medicine is more than the scientific evidence alone, as it also needs to integrate clinical expertise and the patient's preferences.

Often the clinician has the choice between different medical treatments, which have all proved effective in randomized trials, but which have never been compared with one another. Here economic considerations may determine the choice, both for the patient's sake and for the sake of society. *Usually, new drugs are more expensive than those already on the market, and they should not be prescribed unless it has been shown by randomized trials, and preferably by a meta-analysis, that they are better than the old ones.* Unfortunately, there are numerous examples where effective marketing made doctors disregard this principle. New synthetic opiates have been accepted as, allegedly, the risk of addiction was smaller, and new antirheumatic drugs have been preferred to the old ones because they were said to be more powerful and less ulcerogenic, but in these and many other cases it was found later that the assertions were false.

Clinicians in their attempts to keep up-to-date should only rely on unbiased sources such as The Cochrane Library, and as a general rule they should pay no attention to information from advertisements and representatives from drug firms. One would never expect a car dealer to admit that his car is more expensive, but no better, than those of the competitors, and, similarly, a doctor cannot possibly expect to be told by the agent of a pharmaceutical company that there is no reliable evidence that his new drug is better than other, cheaper ones already on the market. Doctors can be quite naïve, however, and flawed industry-sponsored drug trials and drug marketing are very effective, partly because it often involves financial and other benefits to doctors, particularly to opinion leaders. Therefore, many drugs that are 5–10 times more expensive than their competitors are those that are most widely used, although it is unknown whether they are any better. Actually, in some cases, it was shown later in trials that were publicly funded that these expensive drugs were not better, for instance a calcium channel blocker for hypertension[186] and so-called 'atypical' antipsychotic drugs for schizophrenia.[187,188] Other drugs are in common use that are not only more expensive, but also worse than their competitors. This state of affairs, which from an ethical and societal point of view is indefensible, of course, has recently received a lot of attention from medical journal editors and others, for instance in a number of interesting books with rather telling titles.[49,168,189–193]

7
Medicine and the Humanities

Surely there exists no wider gulf, nor more stubborn resistance to bridging it, than that which for centuries has separated science and humanities in medicine. That this should be so in medicine is a remarkable paradox, for medicine, after all, is by its very nature a human science, historically perhaps the very first human science.

Engel[194]

There is a strong tendency to-day to identify knowledge with natural science. But, as two wars have made us painfully aware, natural science can only tell us the means, not how these means ought to be used ... The study of science must therefore be supplemented by a study of the right way of using the knowledge it provides.

Ewing[195]

The four components of clinical reasoning

Traditionally, a distinction is made between science and the humanities. Natural scientists are observers of Nature, whereas their counterparts from the humanities take an interest in human feelings and endeavour to understand and interpret all the different ways in which human beings express themselves. Scientists seek the causes of the phenomena they observe and try to establish the laws of Nature, whereas humanists, as we shall call them, are concerned with reasons rather than causes.[13]

It is one of the fascinations of clinical medicine that it belongs to both these two worlds. The clinician uses the scientific approach when she regards

Table 7.1   The four components of the basis of clinical decisions.

Scientific thinking

1) The deductive component
  Inferences from theoretical knowledge about diseases and disease mechanisms.
2) The empirical component
  Inferences from experience gained from the study of previous patients.
  Uncontrolled experience.
  Controlled experience.

Humanistic thinking

3) The empathic-hermeneutic component
  Inferences from an understanding of the patient as a fellow human being.
4) The ethical component
  Inferences from ethical norms.

---

her patient's disease as an objective phenomenon to be observed, explained and perhaps remedied, but at the same time she adopts a humanistic approach seeing her patient as a human being whose situation she must try to understand. This chapter deals with the humanistic approach, but before we proceed to that topic we shall take a comprehensive view of the structure of clinical reasoning (Table 7.1).

In the preceding parts of this book I have tried to analyse clinical thinking from a scientific point of view and have pointed out that scientific reasoning has two components. Firstly, the decision about the diagnosis or the decision to institute a particular treatment may be the result of theoretical considerations. This means that the clinician tries to deduce from her theoretical knowledge of the structure and functions of the human organism what is the patient's diagnosis and what treatment will have the desired effect. This is the deductive component of scientific reasoning. Secondly, the diagnostic or therapeutic decision may be based on experience, i.e. uncontrolled or controlled experience that was gained in the past by the examination or treatment of similar patients. This is the empirical component of scientific reasoning.

I shall not repeat the discussion of the relative merits of these types of reasoning, but only recapitulate that deductions from theoretical knowledge can rarely be trusted due to the complexity of the functions of the human organism, and that, for an number of reasons, uncontrolled experience is also unreliable (Chapter 5). Therefore, our decisions must, as far as possible, be based on controlled experience, especially studies of the value of diagnostic tests, using the direct method (Chapter 4), and randomized clinical trials (Chapter 6).

In this chapter I shall focus on the humanistic approach to clinical decision-making, which also has two components that I shall label the empathic-hermeneutic component and the ethical component.

The empathic-hermeneutic component

Disease or illness, according to the humanistic approach, is the way in which the individual patient experiences and interprets the different symptoms in the context of her own life. This experience often involves anxiety and suffering, and the clinical decision-maker must try to understand what the patient really feels. Therefore, empathy, which is the ability to see oneself in somebody else's situation, is an important clinical concept.

In some cases empathic understanding is quite straightforward. Consider, for instance, a male middle-aged consultant who in the outpatient department sees a male, middle-aged academic who lives in the same part of the town. Then doctor and patient have much the same background, and, probably, they will find it very easy to understand each other.

But perhaps the next patient seen by this consultant is a young female immigrant from Turkey who tells him about her problems. There is no language problem at all as her English is fluent, but empathy fails, as the consultant knows too little about her background to be able to see the situation from her point of view. If he had had Turkish friends or had spent some time in a Turkish village, or if he had just read some books about Turkish family life, he would have been in a better position. The point is that empathy requires knowledge, and it was lacking in this case. This knowledge, which is needed to understand another person from that person's perspective, is called *hermeneutic knowledge* (from Greek *hermeneutike* = art of interpretation).

Empathy, however, may fail for other reasons than lack of knowledge about a patient's cultural background. Few doctors, for instance, have experienced what it means to receive a diagnosis of incurable cancer, or to be admitted to hospital due to sudden and unexpected praecordial pain, and very few have tried to live their lives as dialysis patients or to have a permanent ileostomy. Doctors who see many such patients may gradually acquire the necessary hermeneutic knowledge, but there is a shortcut that is not sufficiently appreciated. Knowledge, including hermeneutic knowledge, can be committed to writing and communicated to others.

A colleague found it difficult to talk to incurably ill cancer patients. He felt that these patients, who knew they would die within a limited period of time, were living in a world of their own which he could not penetrate. Then he read

Kübler-Ross' book 'On Death and Dying'[196] which reports what this author learnt by interviewing 200 incurable cancer patients at regular intervals. She quotes what the patients told her, often using their own words, and she describes the stages of denial, anger, bargaining, depression and, finally, acceptance. After having spent a few hours reading this small book, the colleague found it much easier to understand his patients, e.g. the patient who seemed to have 'forgotten' what she had been told about her prognosis and was now busy planning her life several years ahead, the patient who during previous visits had been very composed, but now met everybody with anger and accusations, and the patient who said that she was willing to die if only once more, sitting in her garden, she could experience the coming of spring.

Kübler-Ross' book may be regarded as an early example of a qualitative study or, as it ought to be called, a hermeneutic study, and I shall illustrate this kind of research by two other examples. A Danish doctor interviewed a number of patients who had made an appointment with their general practitioner and, after the visits had taken place, she interviewed the doctors and repeated the interviews of the patients.[197] The general impression was a positive one, of patients trusting their doctors and of doctors trying to understand their patients, but the communication between them was by no means perfect. The general practitioners often thought that they were expected to write a prescription when, in fact, the patients' primary wish was not treatment, but just an explanation of their symptoms.

Doctors, of course, provide such explanations, but when they do, they tend to talk about anatomical lesions and physiological malfunction and that does not satisfy the patients who search for the cause in their daily lives. Many misunderstandings could be avoided if doctors, at the beginning of each consultation, spent a little more time letting their patients talk freely about their illness, the way the symptoms affect their daily lives, their fears for the future and what they themselves believe caused the illness. It is important that the history is as complete as possible, but too much essential information is lost if the questioning is reduced to a series of brief questions (Where does it hurt? Does the pain radiate? In what direction?). The scientific approach invites the systematic collection of well-defined data, whereas the humanistic approach requires that the patient's illness is seen in the context of the patient's life. Lack of time should not be a reason for not listening to the patient, as careful listening in the beginning very likely saves time in the end.

Interest in hermeneutic research is on the increase, especially among nurses, but unfortunately the results are rarely published in the ordinary medical journals. In one study a nurse focussed on patients with chronic renal disease.[198] She interviewed patients receiving haemodialysis either in hospital or in their own homes, patients waiting for a donor kidney, patients who had received one, and patients who had suffered rejection of the graft. These categories of patients experienced their situation very differently, and the study communicates essential hermeneutic knowledge that it may take years to acquire working at a nephrology unit.

The methods used in such studies were first developed by anthropologists and sociologists.[199] They differ from conventional scientific ones in a number of respects, e.g. the selection of patients, the choice of interview technique and the analysis of the results, but they also require meticulous planning, a detailed protocol and stringent reasoning.

The ethical component

Scientific reasoning guided by empathic understanding is an essential part of clinical decision-making, but it has its limitations. Scientists can answer questions like these: 'What *is* the patient's diagnosis?', 'What *can* we do?' or 'What *are* the outcomes of these treatments in this randomized trial? But they cannot tell us what we *ought* to do in a particular situation. It is impossible to make this jump from the 'is' and the 'can' of the world of science and technology to the 'ought' of clinical practice without including a value judgment. We must decide whether the consequences of our actions are good or bad and whether the actions themselves are acceptable, and such value judgments belong to the sphere of ethics. Therefore, clinical decision-making always has an ethical component.

Very often the value judgment that determines the decision is so uncontroversial that it is not noted. It is, for instance, a fact that most patients who have developed a cataract and are almost blind will regain their faculty of vision when the lens is removed and replaced by glasses, and it is tempting to conclude from this statement that therefore, we ought to remove the lens in patients with this disease, but this conclusion cannot be deduced from the facts alone. It also depends on the value judgment that it is better to see than to be blind. If we make the absurd assumption that the opposite were true, it would of course be wrong to do this operation.

In other cases the situation is less simple. There are, for instance, three different treatments of hyperthyroidism, the popularities of which have varied over the years: long-term treatment with antithyroid drugs, subtotal thyroidectomy and treatment with radioactive iodine. The decision how to treat these patients depends, among other things, on their age, the size of the goitre and the possibility of pregnancy, and, obviously, we must pay great attention to the results of follow-up studies, preferably in the form of randomized trials. These trials, however, do not provide the final answer. We must also make complex value judgments balancing the risk of post-operative vocal cord paralysis against the possible harms of antithyroid drugs and the possibility of myxoedema following treatment with radioactive iodine. These values cannot be determined once and for all, as they depend on the preferences of the individual patient.

Some doctors seem to hold the view that clinical medicine is a scientific discipline, and that medical ethics is no more than a set of rules that must be respected when we are dealing with patients. They have missed the point which was first made by the philosopher David Hume: You can never derive an 'ought' from an 'is'. All clinical decisions require value judgments and the ethical component must never be overlooked.

Three kinds of norms

We use the words *ethics* and *moral philosophy* synonymously, which is defensible from an etymological point of view, as Greek *ethos* and Latin *mores* originally had the same meaning (habits or customs). Ethics concern what we ought to do and what is good, but it is worth noticing that these (and similar) normative words are also used in non-ethical (non-moral) contexts. Confusion arises when we overlook the distinction between technical, legal and ethical norms.

Technical norms tell us what is good, or effective, for reaching certain pre-defined goals, regardless of the moral goodness of those goals. Thus, a good knife is a sharp knife, and a good revolver is one that makes you hit the bull's eye. Defiance of technical norms is an invitation to practical difficulties as we may not, for instance, be able to cut what we want to cut with a blunt knife, or to hit what we want to hit with a bad revolver. Technical norms are established by means of scientific methods and in many contexts they may also be termed scientific norms. A good or effective antineoplastic drug is one that, according to the results of randomized trials, increases the survival, but it may also cause harms that reduce the patient's quality of life.

Legal norms determine what we may do and may not do according to the law, and if we defy those norms we may be punished. A gynaecologist may feel that it is morally justified to do an abortion, but, if it is illegal in that situation, she may run into serious trouble.

Ethical or moral norms differ from the other two types as they tell us which actions and which consequences are good in themselves (intrinsically good), and those who violate these norms will be met with the moral indignation of others or suffer a guilty conscience. Different people may accept different norms, but most of us agree that it is intrinsically good to speak the truth and to help other people, and that pain and suffering are intrinsically bad. If we state that we ought to institute a certain treatment in order to ensure the patient a good quality of life, we are also using the word *good* in its ethical sense, as a person's quality of life is good or bad in itself.

It is important not to mix up these three kinds of norms, although it is easy to do so as the same statement may sometimes be interpreted in different ways. The sentence: 'You ought not give this young girl those contraceptive pills' may refer to a legal norm (i.e. it is forbidden to do so, according to the law, without the parents' consent), a technical norm (i.e. scientific studies have shown that these pills cause more harms than other pills) or an ethical norm (i.e. if you do it you are acting immorally).

Medical doctors sometimes find it difficult to distinguish between scientific (technical) and ethical norms. A transplantation surgeon, for instance, once said that there was no ethical problem, if he had only one organ at his disposal, but two patients who needed one. He would just give the organ to that patient who would be ensured the best prognosis. Consequently, if he had had two female patients, one who was childless and one who had two children, he would presumably have disregarded that fact, but by doing so he would have taken the ethical stance that being responsible for small children is ethically irrelevant.

Lawyers and some ethicists who focus on individual rights, on their part, tend not to distinguish too sharply between ethical and legal norms. It is often seen, especially in American literature on medical ethics, that ethical problems from clinical practice are reduced to a legal discussion of patients' rights.

The foundation of health care ethics

For a period of three months the doctors from the medical department of a large hospital were asked to make a note each time they faced a significant ethical problem, i.e. a situation where they were in doubt which decision to make or suspected that some of their colleagues might have decided differently. During those three months 426 patients were admitted to the department and in 25% of these cases the doctors recorded one or more such problems.[200]

This example illustrates well the importance of ethical reasoning in clinical practice, and it is quite justified that medical ethics is now being recognized as an academic discipline in its own right. However, it is also important to realize that ethical norms vary in different parts of the world and that medical ethics must be taught differently in different countries. Medical ethics is not international as are the scientific medical disciplines. Admittedly, a number of international organizations have issued ethical declarations on a variety of medical topics, but they rarely offer much guidance in the concrete case. They may be helpful in the sense that they establish certain international guidelines, but at best they represent 'the smallest common denominator' for the norms in different societies, and at worst they are dominated by the norms of one particular culture.

This book is intended for an international readership, and therefore I shall stress the structure of ethical reasoning rather than the solution of the problems. I do not, however, wish to conceal my own ethical intuitions, and I shall describe openly the approach to health care ethics to which I am committed. It is, I believe, the approach that prevails in those European countries that have a public health service (such as the Nordic countries and the UK) and those that seek the same general goal by means of some sort of universal health insurance scheme. The ethical basis of the health services in these countries is best described by means of three principles:

1. *The Samaritan principle,* i.e. the obligation of all citizens to help each other in case of illness.

2. *The principle of distributive justice,* i.e. the obligation to ensure a just distribution of the limited resources of the health service.

3. *The principle of autonomy,* i.e. the obligation to respect the individual right to self-determination.

The *Samaritan principle* must be regarded as a fundamental ethical principle in our part of the world, as health services which offer free hospital treatment to everybody would make no sense if people did not accept this obligation. The principle stresses our mutual obligations and it may therefore be seen as a special case of the Golden Rule 'to do unto others as you would have them do unto you'.[201] This idea of reciprocity is recognized not only in the Christian tradition, but also by many other cultures and religions. In modern societies with a public health care system the individual citizens may be said to fulfil their Samaritan duty by paying for the health service, which then employs professional Samaritans, i.e. doctors, nurses, etc., to carry out the work.

The resources of any health service, however, are limited and therefore it is also necessary to accept a principle of distributive justice or, as it was once said, to ensure 'that everybody gets a fair share of the national health cake'. Thirdly, the countries in question are democratic, and therefore the Samaritan activities of the health service must be carried out in such a way that due respect is paid to individual autonomy.

None of these principles should be accepted at face value. The Golden Rule has many interpretations, the concept of justice is a controversial topic, and respect for autonomy, which we shall discuss below, has been understood differently by different philosophers. However, the principles provide a starting point for our ethical deliberations, and they reveal the difference between health care ethics in, for instance, Europe and the United States. American ethicists also formulate basic principles, but usually the principle of autonomy comes first, and the formulation of the Samaritan principle (which they call the principle of beneficence) is much weaker. Once it was stated in an ethical declaration that 'all persons have some moral obligation to benefit others, to some degree, perhaps especially those who are in need', and, according to that view, the goal of the public health care system is limited to ensuring 'universal access to an acceptable, decent minimum of basic health care'.[202,203] One should not, however, draw too sharp a line between North American and European health care ethics. Libertarian norms, like the American ones, are gaining ground in Europe, the Canadian norms seem closer to those in Europe than those in the United States, and in the United States there are many people who see the need for health service reforms.

The structure of ethical reasoning

Some doctors seem to think that it is a futile exercise to discuss ethical problems, as, in the last resort, moral statements express no more than the feelings of the speaker. This view of ethics (which moral philosophers call emotivism) is fallacious, as ethical problems, just like scientific ones, can be subjected to a logical analysis. First of all, ethical reasoning must be consistent, which means that like cases must be treated alike, or, to put it differently, that a person who decides to do one thing in one situation and another thing in another situation must be able to state the ethically relevant difference. A doctor once argued that the moment of conception marks the beginning of a human life, that the wilful interruption of a human life is murder, and that, consequently, abortion amounts to murder; but this doctor also said that he accepted contraception by means of an intrauterine device. He obviously felt intuitively that the two situations differed, but he ought to have realized that his argument against abortion also applied to that form of contraception.

It would also be most unfortunate if ethics committees, including those that review medical research, regarded ethics as a question of personal feelings. Their answers to ethical problems may not be true or false in any objective sense, but they must have subjected them to a thorough analysis. It is quite justified to accuse the members of an ethics committee of incompetence if they do not act consistently and are unable to justify their decisions rationally.

The ethical decision process is a stepwise procedure. The very first step is the recognition of the problem, and it cannot be taken for granted that all doctors are skilful in this respect. The project where the staff at a medical department were asked to record all significant ethical problems illustrated that it requires training. Prior to the study the doctors had had no particular interest in medical ethics and at the beginning they saw very few problems, but gradually they learnt to recognize the ethical component of their decisions. It is one of the most important goals of the teaching of medical ethics to undergraduates that they learn to detect those ethical problems which they are likely to face as medical practitioners, so that they do not, as the transplantation surgeon mentioned above, overlook the ethical component of their decisions.

The recognition of an ethical problem is tantamount to the recognition of a conflict between different ethical considerations, but usually we intuitively feel what is right and wrong and what would be the best decision. This initial intuition will reflect our own ethical norms, the norms of the society in which we live, as well as generally accepted professional norms. We can no longer say that the practice of medicine must be regarded as a vocation to help others, but the driving force behind all clinical decisions must still be the wish to relieve human suffering and to combine technical expertise with true compassion and understanding. The ethical and the empathic components of the clinical decision process cannot be separated. A clinician once recommended the use of the *uncle test*, by which he meant that the doctor should imagine that the patient was a dear uncle of hers. Whenever she faced an ethical problem, she should ask the following question: How would I like my uncle's doctor to act in this situation? The uncle test seems preferable to a spouse, child or parent test, as it ensures that the decision-maker has warm feelings, but is not so emotionally involved that she cannot think rationally.

However, the immediate intuition and the 'uncle test' will not provide adequate answers to complex ethical dilemmas. It is necessary to proceed with a rational analysis of the problem at hand, including both factual and ethical considerations.

Assessment of the facts of the case

When different people disagree about the answer to an ethical problem it will often be found that their ethical attitudes are much the same, but that their assessment of the facts differ. The factual basis of the problem must, in this connection, be interpreted very broadly, as it comprises not only the assessment of the clinical data and the patient's situation, but also the assessment of the prognosis and the probable outcome of different decisions. Imagine, for instance, the situation where one doctor recommends resuscitation of a patient who has suffered a stroke whereas a colleague finds that the patient should be allowed to die. It is possible that these colleagues have similar ethical norms, but that their assessment differed as regards the patient's condition, the likely prognosis after resuscitation and the wishes of the relatives.

Participants in ethical debates often appeal to the so-called slippery slope argument. They may find that some action is morally acceptable here and now, but hold that it should not be allowed, as they fear that it would lead to other practices that they regard as morally unacceptable. Some people, for instance, argue that active euthanasia may be morally acceptable in some terminal cancer cases, but that it should not be legalized as it might lead to euthanasia in other situations where it is quite unacceptable. In such cases the assessment of the consequences, if they occur, is an ethical problem, but the assessment of the likelihood that they will occur is a factual problem.

Consequential considerations

Consequential considerations play a very important role in the ethical decision process. They serve to compare the 'goodness' of the consequences of different actions, and that is not always easy to do.

In our daily lives there are many situations where we have the choice between different decisions, and then we usually start by considering the consequences for particular individuals, especially members of our family, friends and colleagues. These are the *person-orientated consequential considerations*. Often, however, we must think further than that. We must, for instance, take into account the general consequences for other people if we do not pay our income tax as required or if we pollute the environment unnecessarily. In such cases it is tempting to make the excuse that the consequences of one's own action are insignificant in a larger perspective, but then one may generalize the consequential consideration and ask: What would the general consequences be if everybody acted that way under similar circumstances? This question serves as a guide to the *universal consequential considerations.*

The ethics of the doctor–patient relationship can be described in much the same way. The clinician sees it as her primary goal to do the best for her patient and, if she has the choice between different actions, she must try to decide which one is likely to have the best consequences in that particular case. These patient-orientated consequential considerations may be quite complicated, as they require not only that she compares the goodness of all possible outcomes, but also that she assesses the probability that these outcomes will occur. A very good consequence (curing the patient) may counterbalance a very bad consequence (a serious complication) if the probability of the former is sufficiently high and that of the latter sufficiently small. The assessment of the goodness of a consequence is a value judgment and as such it belongs to the realm of ethics, whereas the assessment of the probability requires empirical evidence and belongs to the realm of science.

Statistical decision theorists[8] have suggested that these consequential considerations may be formalized by 'measuring' the goodness or *utility* (U) of the different consequences on an interval scale from zero to one. Then, if we know the probability of these consequences, it becomes possible to calculate the expected utility, $\Sigma(P \times U)$, of each decision, i.e. the average 'amount of goodness' produced by that decision. This procedure illustrates well the logic of consequential considerations, but obviously it cannot be used in practice. The goodness of a consequence for a particular person cannot be measured in centimetres or any other interval scale.

Other people-orientated considerations may also be needed, as the clinician may have to assess the consequences for the patient's relatives and sometimes also the consequences for herself. Apart from that, universal considerations may be required to assess the consequences for the health service and for future patients. I shall illustrate the complexity of these consequential considerations by means of some examples, but first I shall consider a very different type of ethical considerations.

Deontological considerations

Some moral philosophers, who call themselves utilitarians or consequentialists, hold that ethical reasoning is no more than an assessment of consequences, but most people would probably deny that. They would not accept that the end always justifies the means, as they believe that some actions, regardless of the consequences, are more acceptable than others from an ethical point of view.

Therefore, it is necessary to take into account a very different type of ethical consideration, which is usually called *deontological* (from Greek *deon* = duty) although it does not only concern our duties, but also our rights. The deontological way of thinking is well illustrated by the Ten Commandments in the Old Testament. One of the commandments reads: Thou shalt not steal! It does not say that it is forbidden, if the consequences are bad, but that it is quite permissible if (as in the case of Robin Hood) the consequences are good. It is the act of stealing as such that is objectionable from a moral point of view.

The most important deontological principles in medical ethics are the duties to respect the patient's autonomy, to preserve life, to speak the truth, to respect the patient's dignity and to maintain confidentiality. All these duties are important, but in spite of that we must realize that it is difficult to imagine a deontological principle that is absolute. Life must be preserved by active treatment, except when the quality of that life is very low, and the maintenance of confidentiality is essential, except for those rare cases where the interests of society or other individuals must take priority. Therefore, moral duties are said to be *prima facie* duties which means that they are morally binding except in those cases where other (deontological or consequential) considerations have greater weight.

The ethical decision

Finally, the clinical decision-maker must decide which action is the most acceptable one from an ethical point of view, and in some cases the different kinds of considerations have clarified the situation to such an extent that she is in no doubt what to do. In other cases, however, the dilemma is not solved that easily. The clinician feels that she has taken into account all the important consequential and deontological considerations and she realizes that, on balance, they call for one particular decision, but unfortunately she also feels that she cannot reconcile that conclusion with her ethical intuition and basic ethical beliefs. In that case she can do no more than rethink the problem once again and search her mind for those ethical considerations which determined her intuition, and if she finds none, she may well experience that during the analytic process her intuition gradually changes. However, ethical dilemmas do not always have an unequivocal solution. Experienced clinicians, facing a difficult decision, sometimes know in advance that, whatever they do, they will be left with a guilty conscience.

I do not suggest, of course, that the clinician should always sit down and make a list of all the different consequential and deontological considerations, although sometimes it might not be a bad idea. Most of the ethical problems which medical practitioners face in ordinary clinical practice are not unique, and they will have adopted a policy of their own, as regards, for instance, the information of cancer patients or the treatment of those who are terminally ill. Routine, however, should never prevail to such an extent that we forget that we are faced with an ethical problem and that each patient is unique.

It is also important, especially at hospitals in a public health service, that clinical decisions do not depend too much on the ethical norms of one particular doctor. Patients rarely choose their doctors themselves, and even when they do, they cannot know very much about their ethical norms. Therefore, before they make the decisions, doctors ought to discuss all major ethical problems, both with their colleagues and with those nurses who know the patient well. Such conferences may reveal that the doctor presenting a problem has overlooked some important ethical consideration, and, in the long run, the discussions will promote a harmonization of the ethical norms in that particular department.

Quality of life

The most important consequential considerations are, of course, the patient-orientated ones, which aim at choosing that decision which has the best consequences for the patient. The meaning of the word 'best' in this context is rather uncontroversial if it is simply a question of curing the patient or of removing unpleasant symptoms, and the risk of treatment complications is very small, but in other contexts it is not so simple to decide what is good and what is not so good, and it is in such cases that it has become fashionable to talk about quality of life.

The expression 'quality of life' is used in different ways, and it is never defined in exact terms. Most often, it denotes something subjective, and in that sense it is used in much the same way as decision theorists use the word utility and moral philosophers previously talked about happiness. At that time the utilitarian philosopher, Jeremy Bentham, tried to develop what he called a felicific calculus in order to measure happiness, and that idea, which later was completely abandoned by moral philosophers, has now been revived by those who believe that it possible to measure the utility of different decisions or the patients' subjective quality of life on some interval scale. I shall not discuss the methods that have been suggested, as none of them are practicable.

In a medical context we face the additional conceptual problem that we should not concern ourselves with the patient's subjective quality of life as such, but only with her health-related quality of life. It is a medical problem if the reduction of a patient's quality of life is caused by her illness, but not if it is caused by family trouble or problems at work.

Quality of life is also sometimes used in an objective sense as something that can be observed, and, within limits, that is a reasonable idea. Human beings may differ, but presumably we should all feel that our subjective quality of life was reduced if arthritic changes made it difficult for us to climb stairs, dress or take a bath, or if a cataract prevented us from reading the morning paper or looking at TV. Therefore, it is very important both in everyday clinical practice and for research purposes that all such disabilities are recorded and perhaps quantified by means of simple rating scales, but it is much less obvious that it should be possible to combine the observations and to calculate some sort of objective quality of life score. Usually, the weighting of the individual items is quite arbitrary, and the validity of the resulting score remains a matter of belief. Even such composite scales that the authors claim to have 'validated' usually cannot stand up to a logical analysis.

Thus, quality of life measurements remain a dubious affair, but we should, of course, listen to our patients when they tell us about their lives and we should try to take a comprehensive view of their clinical condition. Such informal judgments play an important role in the decision process, and sometimes we find that there is little agreement between the quality of life as it is experienced by the patient herself and our assessment of the patient's quality of life. We see some patients who appear to be in a very poor state, but still claim that they are very happy. They seem to have reduced their expectations of life and to have accepted their condition. Others complain that their lives are completely ruined by some symptom or disability that from the doctor's point of view seems rather trivial. They seem to have expected a life devoid of problems of any kind.

Up to now we have only considered the quality of life at a given moment in time, but clinicians also wish to predict their patient's condition in the years to come. Decision theorists have tried to formalize such predictions, and their approach has provoked considerable debate. They suggest that doctors should calculate the number of quality-adjusted life years or QALYs, i.e. the number of years that a patient is expected to live multiplied by her quality of life (measured on a scale from zero to one). This product is thought to represent the 'amount of quality of life' that the patient is expected to accumulate during the remaining part of her life. If different treatments are available, one should calculate the number of QALYs that is produced by each of these, and then choose the one that from this point of view ensures the best prognosis. I have already mentioned that it is impossible to measure quality of life on an interval scale, but apart from that the idea is conceptually bizarre, as it is assumed that it is as good to live one year with a quality of life of one as to live 10 years with a quality of life of 0.1.

Nevertheless, it is important that clinicians take an interest in the age-old concept of 'a good life'. The majority will probably say that they would like to keep fit and live to a great age (without specifying what they mean by that) and then die suddenly. They fear above anything else that they will grow senile and helpless, so that they will have to spend the last part of their life in a nursing home. We often say, when somebody dies whom we knew well, that this person had a good life except for the last few years, which she would have been better without. Epidemiologists regularly report that a large number of sudden deaths from myocardial infarction, mostly among elderly people, could have been prevented if people changed their lifestyle in one way or another, and their findings are widely publicized through the media. They forget to tell us that some of these sudden deaths forestalled an end to life that very few people would wish for themselves.

Autonomy and paternalism

Autonomy and paternalism are key concepts in medical ethics. An autonomous decision is a decision which is made after due consideration without external coercion, and an autonomous person is a person who is able to make such decisions. In contrast, a non-autonomous or incompetent person is someone who, for some reason or other, is unable to do so. We have already mentioned the principle of autonomy, which for all practical purposes is interpreted as the duty to respect the individual right to self-determination.

Moral philosophers use different definitions of paternalism, but here we shall say that a person A acts paternalistically towards another person B, when A – with or without B's consent – chooses that decision that she believes has the best consequences for B. Using this definition, a distinction may be made between three forms of paternalism: genuine, solicited and unsolicited paternalism.

Genuine paternalism is paternalistic action towards non-autonomous people, and the typical example is the father (*pater*) who imposes his will on his small child 'because daddy knows best'. But it is not only children who must be regarded as non-autonomous. Doctors see patients who are unconscious, delirious because of a high temperature, psychotic or severely mentally handicapped, and in all such cases there is no doubt that paternalistic action is morally required.

Solicited paternalism is paternalistic action towards autonomous patients who have said that they have no wish to take part in the decision process but wish to leave the decisions to the doctor. If the wish has been expressed unambiguously, this type of paternalism is also morally acceptable.

Unsolicited paternalism is paternalistic action towards autonomous patients without their consent, i.e. those situations where a doctor institutes diagnostic procedures or treatments without having consulted the patient in advance. Doctors should of course always make up their mind which decisions will serve their patients' interests best, but that does not necessarily imply that those decisions should be implemented. To use the terminology that was introduced above, the patient-orientated consequential considerations are subject to the deontological constraint that the patient's autonomy must be respected.

Today it is generally agreed that, as a general rule, unsolicited paternalism is morally unacceptable. There can be little doubt that previously most doctors indulged too much in unsolicited paternalism, and that today most patients expect that their autonomy is respected. However, it must also be realized that there is no sharp distinction between autonomy and non-autonomy, and that, consequently, there is a grey zone between genuine and unsolicited paternalism. Paediatricians must take into account the degree of maturity of the individual child, psychiatrists face particularly difficult ethical and legal problems when they consider treatment against the patient's own wish, and all other clinicians see numerous borderline cases where it is a matter of judgment whether or not paternalistic action is justified.

In some cases one may even talk about a selective loss of autonomy. Many drug addicts must be regarded as fully autonomous in many respects, but, due to their physical dependence on the drugs, those actions that are related to the abuse cannot be regarded as autonomous. Their right to self-determination must be respected in many situations, but genuine paternalism may be required when the decisions concern the addictive behaviour. Therapists sometimes talk about establishing 'contracts' with addicts, and that may be reasonable from a pedagogical point of view, but these contracts do not have the same moral status as ordinary contracts between autonomous persons.

I have selected below a number of illustrative examples that are meant to illustrate important aspects of the structure of ethical reasoning. I do not seek to promote any particular ethical views, although I shall not try to conceal my own ethical attitudes.

Clinical examples

Example 1

A 55-year-old woman has felt a dull pain below the right costal margin and is referred to hospital by her general practitioner. Ultrasonically guided biopsies revealed metastases from an adenocarcinoma in both liver lobes. It is concluded that there is no effective treatment. What should the patient be told? This example will be used to illustrate some important aspects of ethical reasoning. The considerations vary from case to case, but as a starting point it is often useful to ask the following three questions:

1. Which decision will have the best consequences for my patient? This is the patient-orientated consequential consideration mentioned above, and it is related to the Samaritan principle of health care ethics.

2. What would the general consequences be if all doctors acted in that way under similar circumstances? This is the universal consequential consideration, and one of the examples below will illustrate the connection between this question and the principle of justice.

3. Is my patient autonomous, and, if so, do I respect my patient's right to self-determination? This is a deontological consideration, which corresponds to the principle of autonomy.

As regards the first of these questions, most doctors would probably say that in this case it is best for the patient to be informed about the diagnosis and prognosis. They will argue that, in the long run, it will not be possible to conceal the diagnosis from her, and that it will be much easier to support her if she is told the truth from the start. Apart from that there may be many things of a practical nature which she would wish to settle while there is still time.

Then, according to the second question, we should ask ourselves what would happen if all doctors concealed the diagnosis from cancer patients, and again we must conclude that, in general, patients ought to be told the truth. When patients, as in this case, are going to die from their disease, the diagnosis will be revealed sooner or later, and it would become general knowledge that doctors lie. That might cause lack of trust in the medical profession, and it might have the secondary effect that patients with chronic benign diseases suffered unnecessarily. They would not believe the doctor who told them quite truthfully that their disease was not malignant. Further, we must consider those patients who are cured from their cancer, e.g. patients with a colonic cancer who are cured by a colonic resection. If they were never told that they had had a cancer, people would only hear about those cancer patients who died, and the population would be led to believe that cancer is always incurable. These considerations are not theoretical, as we experienced these effects when doctors, about 50 years ago, rarely told their patients the true diagnosis.

The answer to the third question points in the same direction. Withholding the information would be a violation of the patient's autonomy, as the patient cannot decide what to do with the limited rest of her life if she is not adequately informed.

Some readers will disagree with my answers to the three questions. A large survey has shown that almost all Northern European and North American doctors would tell such a patient the truth, but that most doctors in Southern Europe and especially Eastern Europe would conceal the diagnosis and prognosis.[204] This difference must reflect differences as regards both ethical norms and factual beliefs. Obviously, doctors in Southern and Eastern Europe do not stress the third deontological consideration as much as their Northern European colleagues do today, but they must also believe, as Northern European doctors did some decades ago, that telling the truth would cause greater psychological distress. This survey also showed that Southern and Eastern European doctors always told the spouse the full truth, for which reason their information policy will not have all those general effects which were recorded as the answer to the second question.

Obviously, the policy of openness does not imply that patients should just be told the crude facts. The information must be part of a dialogue where the clinician feels her way, notices the patient's reaction, finds out how much the patient wishes to know at that particular moment, and offers further consultations. In other words, adequate information presupposes empathic understanding. When, for instance, the doctor uses the word cancer, she must be aware of the fact that it will be interpreted very differently by different patients. One patient may have known somebody who was completely cured while somebody else may have witnessed one of those tragic cases where the disease was particularly protracted and painful.

Example 2

An 84-year-old man is referred to hospital because of a slight anginal pain, and a chest X-ray reveals a shadow that, probably, is caused by a cancer that, as yet, has produced no symptoms. The patient's general condition precludes surgical intervention. What should this patient be told?

Most doctors who are told about this case seem to agree that it was unfortunate that this somewhat unnecessary X-ray picture was ever taken, implying that it would be best for the patient to remain ignorant of this finding. But that which is best is not always right and some colleagues have argued that the principle of autonomy must be upheld and that the patient must be told.

This is a real case and the clinician in charge applied the uncle test (p. 158). She argued that her imaginary, very sensible 84-year-old uncle would be well aware of the fact that he would not live forever. He would by that time have drawn up a will (if he wanted to make one) and he enjoyed each day. Why should one pester the life of the dear old uncle with this information? She also argued (not quite convincingly) that withholding the information was not a violation of autonomy, but an example of what she called 'implicit solicited paternalism', as she was sure that the old man would not have wanted the information, if one had asked him. As a result of these considerations the patient was not told anything, but the clinician did inform the patient's general practitioner that she had seen a lesion in the lung, which might be a cancer.

I feel that it would be more honest to say that this was a clear-cut example of unsolicited paternalism, where the clinician felt that the patient-orientated consequential consideration took priority over the duty to respect the patient's autonomy. But I have to admit that I sympathize with this colleague who acted out of true compassion. Respect for autonomy requires no warm feelings. It is also relevant to consider the finding that some of the asymptomatic lung cancers that are detected by screening with chest X-rays have a very good prognosis.[205] It is therefore possible that the old man would have died from another cause before he ever knew he had lung cancer.

Example 3

Another old man who also suffered from an incurable cancer had been admitted to hospital. He had not been told about the diagnosis, and before the ward round the nurse asked the doctor to do so. The doctor, who knew the patient well, asked 'Why?', and the nurse replied that it would be best for the patient to know the truth. The point was that the doctor had tried to tell the patient several times, but whenever she approached the topic of his disease he interrupted her and started to talk about something else. Therefore, the doctor had concluded that he did not want to be told. The nurse fully agreed that the doctor's interpretation of the patient's behaviour was correct, but she maintained that the patient should be told for his own sake.

However, according to the principle of autonomy this patient should not be told, because, as an autonomous person, he has the right to refuse information. The nurse was a paternalist, and perhaps she had also, as some people do, twisted the principle of autonomy to mean that people have some sort of duty to be informed and to act autonomously.

Example 4

The Samaritan principle, of course, refers to the parable of the Good Samaritan. A man had been attacked by robbers and left half-dead on the road; then the Samaritan came along, offered first-aid and paid for the man to be cared for at the local inn. This was a case of genuine paternalism, as the word half-dead must mean that the robbed man was unconscious. However, it is tempting to write a modern version of the parable. The man wakes up when he sees the Samaritan and says: 'I do not want your help'. Then the Samaritan would have to make sure that the man was fully conscious and autonomous, and, if that was the case, he would, according to our ethical norms, have to take his donkey and ride on. In Denmark the health authorities admonish doctors that patients have the right to refuse treatment and the British Medical Association has done the same.[17] The deontological consideration takes priority over the consequential ones.

The following case resembles the revised parable. A young woman suffered a large haemorrhage during labour. She is a Jehovah's Witness and she had already made it quite clear, on admission, that she wanted no blood transfusions. She repeated this wish when she started to bleed. The doctors decided not to act against her wish, even when she became unconscious, and the woman died.

This tragic case is interesting from the point of view that it revealed the ambiguity of the ethical norms of the Danish society. A few days later, one of the leading national newspapers wrote in an editorial that the doctors at this hospital had committed murder. The ethical norms in our societies are changing and at a given time both old and new norms prevail. This is one reason why the medical profession, no matter how they act, cannot avoid being met with moral indignation by some members of the community.

Needless to say, the situation would have been entirely different if the bleeding patient had been a child. Then genuinely paternalistic action would have been required, even against the parents' wishes.

Example 5

An old woman, who was physically weak, but not senile, had just had influenza and was severely dehydrated. She said several times that she was tired of life and wished to die. She did not want anything to drink, and she certainly did not want an intravenous drip. The doctor and the staff nurse in unison tried to persuade her that she would feel very much better if she was rehydrated, but she did not change her mind.

In the end the doctor and the nurse decided to overrule her clearly expressed wish. They simply said that it was necessary to put up a drip and did so in spite of her protestations and weak resistance. An observer would have had to conclude that this was a blatant violation of the principle of respect for autonomy, but, after having been rehydrated, the patient regained her zest for life and was very happy when she was discharged from hospital.

It might seem tempting to argue that this was a case of justified genuine paternalism in a temporarily non-autonomous patient, but the woman was autonomous. Furthermore, the doctor and the nurse could not have been sure that the story would have such a happy ending. The patient might have died of old age after some days or weeks, and in that case one would have said that they prolonged her suffering by violating her autonomous wish.

Example 6

A young woman was admitted to hospital suffering from ulcerative colitis. She had had the disease for a long time and had received adequate treatment. Now, she was in a bad condition in spite of that treatment, and a course of corticosteroids had had no appreciable effect. It was concluded that it was necessary to do a total colectomy to save her life, but the patient refused surgical treatment. She said that she did not wish to run the risk of having to have an ileostomy for life. She was told that, probably, it would be possible to restore the normal anatomy by a pouch operation, but that did not make her change her mind. The medical staff used all their powers of persuasion and reminded her of her responsibilities towards her two children, but she still refused. She remained fully conscious and fully aware of her situation. Then, after two weeks, she gave in, saying: 'You leave me no choice', and the colectomy was done. This story also had a happy ending. The patient recovered and fully accepted the treatment she had been given.

One may say that this case presented no serious ethical problem. The doctors gave the patient all the information she needed, and they respected her right to self-determination, as they did not, of course, do the colectomy until the patient had consented. However, we still have to ask to what extent the doctors respected her autonomy. An autonomous decision is a decision that is made without external coercion and in this case the doctors and nurses exposed the patient to maximal psychological pressure. However, most doctors will say, just as the patient did afterwards, that the medical staff acted correctly, and the example shows that good clinical practice often requires an element of paternalism.[206]

Example 7

A middle-aged woman with a duodenal ulcer was seen as an outpatient by a gastroenterologist. At that time this disease could only be treated by lowering the gastric acid production by means of an H_2-receptor antagonist or a proton pump inhibitor, and the latter of these drugs was very expensive. It was known from randomized clinical trials that the cheapest H_2-blocker (cimetidine) healed about 75% of ulcers within four weeks, whereas the proton pump inhibitor healed almost all ulcers. The drug expenses were partly covered by the health service, and it was the policy of that department always to start treatment with cimetidine and to reserve the new drug for that minority of cases which did not respond. This patient did not accept this policy. She had heard about the new drug and demanded that it was prescribed to her from the start.

Consider, once again, the three questions from the first example. From a patient-orientated consequentialist point of view (question 1) there can be no doubt that it would be better, but only marginally so, to receive the new drug from the start. From the deontological point of view (question 3) one might argue that it is the patient's right to decide for herself, but the situation is not quite that simple. Respect for autonomy implies a right to be informed and a right to refuse treatment, but it does not necessarily imply a right to receive any treatment. A person with a common cold, for instance, cannot demand that her doctor writes a prescription for penicillin. But, of course, in this case the woman's wish carries some weight.

The important question is the second one. What would happen to the health service if all doctors started prescribing the expensive drug in such a case? It would obviously cost a lot of money and, since any public health service has a limited budget, it would mean that the money would have to be saved in some other way. This is called the *opportunity cost*, which is the lost opportunities somewhere else in the health service. Doctors employed by a national health service have a duty towards all patients seeking the help of the service, and they are co-responsible for the fair distribution of the limited resources.

The doctor balanced these considerations and decided to maintain that she would only write a prescription for the cheaper drug. She also felt that the patient's wish was somewhat immoral, as those patients who use the facilities of a public health service at no personal cost should respect that the resources must be distributed as fairly as possible.

Example 8

Many of the inhabitants at a nursing home for old people suffered from senile dementia, and from time to time one of them left the home and wandered helplessly round the roads of the neighbourhood. Once, when an old women had done so, the police were contacted, and the officer on duty was willing to send a patrol car round to look for her, but he stressed that they were only allowed to ask her whether she wanted to go home. They would have to respect her right to self-determination.

The nursing home was reasonably well staffed, but they could not prevent such incidents. They could not possibly watch the front door all the time, and in the end they decided to install a combination lock. Those who wished to leave the home would have to press a four-figure number, which would be easy to do for anybody who was not severely demented. That initiative, however, caused a local political uproar. Some politicians said that the old peoples' autonomy had been violated.

Both the policeman's remark and the reaction of the politicians are good examples of absurd misinterpretations of the concepts of autonomy and the right to self-determination. Obviously, the senile inhabitants of the nursing home were not autonomous, and the installation of the combination lock was an act of genuine paternalism. It may be argued from a legal point of view that these people had not been declared incapable of managing their own affairs and that no guardians had been appointed, but, as mentioned above, one should distinguish between law and ethics.

It is peculiar that well-meant and usually quite justified paternalism within the health service causes so much debate when few people object to the compulsory use of safety straps and crash-helmets. Those regulations are good examples of unsolicited paternalism.

Example 9

A 60-year-old man with advanced lung cancer and bone metastases was treated with long-acting opiates orally, but pain relief was quite inadequate. Therefore, a moderate dose of morphine was added to the intravenous drip with some effect. Gradually, the dose was increased and after a few hours the patient was virtually pain-free. The dose was increased no further. Twelve hours later he died.

Most doctors would approve of the treatment of this patient. It could not be excluded, nor proved, that the treatment had shortened his life, but the aim of the treatment was to relieve his distress. The duty to preserve life weighs heavily among the deontological considerations, but, as mentioned earlier, no deontological principle is absolute, and on balance it seems right to have treated the patient in this way.

Then imagine that this patient some months earlier, when he began to feel the pain from the metastases and the diagnosis was first made, had asked his doctor to put an end to his life. He did not want to live through the last few months and his wife agreed with him. The doctor refused as she did not wish to commit a crime, but she also asked herself, 'Should euthanasia be legalized?'

Consider the first of our three standard questions. Would it be best for the patient to die at that time? To help us answer this question we may imagine that the patient on his way home from the doctor had a myocardial infarction and died. In that case both the doctor and the family would probably have said that it was a merciful end to his life, so probably the answer to that question is 'yes'. Then consider the third question. Should we not respect this wish of an autonomous person? As mentioned already (example 7), patients cannot demand any treatment from their doctor and that must include euthanasia, and a doctor cannot be expected to act contrary to her own moral norms. But one might argue that a doctor who approves of euthanasia should be allowed to comply with the patient's wish.

The second question, i.e. the question of the universal consequences, is the one that is most worrying. Legalization would have the effect that all patients with incurable cancer, as well as their relatives, would suffer the additional burden of having to decide whether or not euthanasia was the right solution. Euthanasia is accepted in the Netherlands, and a Dutch woman, whose husband had cancer, once said that she had been given the choice between being her husband's murderer or his torturer!

The slippery slope argument must also be taken into account. The acceptance of euthanasia in incurable cancer might gradually lead to the acceptance of this practice in other categories of patients. There is a Dutch example of euthanasia in the case of a divorced middle-aged woman who had lost both her children and could no longer see the purpose of her life.[207] Possibly, the practice might also be extended to old people who are in a poor state. Such patients sometimes express a wish to die and then explain that they do not wish this for their own sake, but because they are such a burden to their children.

These nine examples serve to illustrate the principles of ethical reasoning in clinical practice, but clinicians, of course, face many other ethical dilemmas. Many of these are well analysed in the publication from the British Medical Association, 'Medical Ethics Today'.[17]

Clinical research ethics

Clinical research is a useful activity in society. People expect that medicine progresses, and that more and more diseases will be amenable to efficient treatment. There is a great need for both basic research and clinical research, including the critical assessment of new and existing diagnostic and therapeutic methods. Each type of research presents ethical problems of its own, but here I shall only consider some of the general principles.

In one respect research ethics differs fundamentally from the ethics of clinical practice. The medical practitioner may sometimes feel the tension between paternalism and respect for autonomy, but if she acts within the grey area between morally justified paternalism and unsolicited paternalism, there is no doubt that she does so to benefit her patient as much as possible. The doctor who violates her patient's right to information and self-determination does so for the patient's own sake.

Clinical researchers also wish to help sick people, but the people they benefit are not primarily those patients who are enrolled in the trials, but future patients. Therefore, the researcher who does not inform the participants of a trial adequately and secures their consent does not act paternalistically; she just violates their autonomy in order to help somebody else. It is the patients themselves who must decide whether or not they wish to behave altruistically. In the past, doctors did not always ask for their patients' consent, but now it is required by the Helsinki Declaration of the World Medical Association[208] and in some countries by law, and it is also required that all research involving humans is approved by a research ethics committee. The structure of the committee system varies from country to country. In many countries it is considered sufficient that each institution establishes a committee of its own, whereas in Denmark a nation-wide independent system of regional committees has been established.

The patients are entitled to both written and verbal information, and it is one of the responsibilities of the ethics committees to ensure that the written information is adequate. Unfortunately, many researchers have great difficulties explaining in plain language without technical terms what their project is about and what it involves from the participants' point of view. The length of the information sheets also varies. In the United States they are very long and detailed as they include a lot of the background documentation, perhaps to protect doctors and drug companies against litigation, whereas they are shorter in Europe, but not necessarily less informative from the patients' point of view.

Research on unconscious, mentally ill or other non-autonomous patients present particular ethical problems, and sometimes consent by proxy is required, but here we shall only discuss research on autonomous persons who can decide for themselves whether or not they wish to participate. When we ask such patients why they wish to take part, we usually get the answer that they do so to benefit future patients. They feel that they themselves benefit from previous research where other patients offered their assistance, and now they accept that it is their turn. This is a very important point as it follows that research that will not benefit future patients is ethically questionable.

Research projects that are methodologically flawed are, of course, always unethical as they will not lead to reliable results, and it ought to be one of the duties of ethics committees to ensure that such projects are never launched. However, there are also those projects that, in spite of the fact that they are methodologically acceptable, are not likely to benefit future patients. Drug firms, for instance, often wish to test new products, which, being chemical analogues of existing drugs, are not likely to be any better than those already marketed. This is, of course, a legitimate enterprise from a commercial point of view, but one may argue that the doctor who asks his patients to participate is betraying their trust. The patients accept on the implicit assumption that they are helping other patients, but usually the only ones who are benefited are, in fact, the drug company and perhaps the doctor who may receive financial support from the company. Such trials also have an opportunity cost, as the patients who volunteer cannot participate in other, more relevant research.

Randomized trials are, of course, also unethical if the problem in question has already be adequately solved by previous trials, and as mentioned before (p. 143) the protocol for a randomized trial should always refer to a systematic review of previous trials. This procedure would also rule out those unnecessary trials that drug firms initiate in order to disseminate knowledge of their product among doctors. These so-called seeding trials are best described as marketing masqueraded as science.

Patients who take part in randomized trials do so on trust. They trust that their doctor will take care of them during the trial and they also trust that the project is worthwhile. Therefore, it is the duty of the doctor who asked them to participate to ensure that the trial is acceptable from a methodological point of view, and she cannot delegate that responsibility to a drug firm. One cannot, of course, expect that all doctors, taking part in a multicentre trial, will possess sufficient knowledge about previous trials, sample size calculations, statistical tests, the handling of drop-outs, etc. to be able to judge for themselves all aspects of the relevance and quality of the trial, but they must make sure that the drug firm has handed over the full responsibility for the trial to an independent, sufficiently qualified steering committee. This committee should be in possession of all the scientific data, and it is their responsibility that the results are published as soon as possible after the conclusion of the trial. The drug firm must not be able to postpone or prevent publication, if the trial did not give the desired result. Clinicians engaged in research should therefore, as a condition for participation, require that they will get access to all the data the trial generates. Without such an agreement, the clinicians cannot live up to their duty towards the patients, which is to ensure that the published article reflects fairly and accurately the data that were collected. Unfortunately, this is not how most drug trials are done. Clinicians usually have very little influence on the analysis and reporting of trials,[169] and a survey showed that it was explicitly stated in half of the trial protocols that the sponsor either owns the data or needs to approve the manuscript.[209]

The sponsoring drug firm has a responsibility of its own, as regards the quality of the project. Therefore, it is both the right and the duty of the company to monitor the running of its own trial at all centres at regular intervals. Doctors involved with a trial do not always do so with sufficient discipline, and there are sad examples of fraud where doctors have 'invented' patients.

It is far more problematic, however, because it is so common, that industry-sponsored drug trials are often designed, analysed and reported in such a way that both the results and the conclusions become biased.[151,161,210–212] It should therefore be a public enterprise to perform those trials that aim to show whether new drugs are better than those in current use. Furthermore, new drugs should not be allowed on the market if they have not been compared with other, similar drugs, but only with placebo, as placebo controlled trials cannot provide the clinicians with the information they need to be able to choose the best drug for their patients.

The majority of clinicians are not actively engaged in research, but they may get involved if they see a patient who takes part in a trial. The patient may have been admitted to hospital as an emergency because of a different disease, or she may have decided to consult her general practitioner for some reason or other. In all such cases the doctor who sees the patient should contact the colleagues running the trial in order to ensure that nothing is done inadvertently which interferes with the protocol. Many clinical researchers have experienced the situation when some patient was lost to their trial because a colleague did not bother to contact them and just told the patient that she had better stop taking the trial medicine for the time being.

8

Critical Reading of Medical Journals

It has come so far that it is difficult to open a medical journal without meeting a misunderstood therapeutic statistical note.

Heiberg[213]

This quotation, which is from 1895, is also relevant today. Statistical methods have become much more advanced, but it has also become much more difficult for the readers to judge whether the data analyses are reliable, as this would require more detail than is commonly presented in medical papers. Even so, readers of medical journals must know enough about research methods and statistics to be able to identify the most common errors and biases.

This chapter is a brief guide to help critical readers not to be misled by methodological flaws, hidden sources of bias and misleading statistical calculations.[12,214] Those who wish to know more about these topics must consult textbooks on research methods, clinical epidemiology and biostatistics.[2,7,9–11,14,16,19] It is also helpful to study guidelines for good reporting of research, e.g. CONSORT for randomized trials,[143] STROBE for observational studies,[215] STARD for diagnostic accuracy studies[84] and PRISMA for systematic reviews and meta-analyses.[216]

Logical analysis of medical papers

The best advice that I can offer the critical reader of a medical paper is to start by analysing its logical structure. Most research projects aim at establishing causal relationships, and it is possible to distinguish between three different approaches:

1. The scientist starts with a putative cause and collects data forward in time on possible effects. The results of the study are conditional probabilities of the type P(effect|cause). Cohort studies are typical examples of this type of reasoning.

2. The scientist starts with an effect and collects data backward in time on possible causes. The results of the study are conditional probabilities of the type P(cause|effect). Some case-control studies are typical examples.

3. The scientist makes all observations at the same time and analyses to what extent different phenomena are associated with one another. He is therefore usually unable to determine the direction of causality. Such studies are called cross-sectional studies.

In the typical *cohort study* one or more groups of persons who fulfil a well-defined set of criteria are selected and are then observed for a period of time. These groups of people are also called *cohorts* (from Latin *cohors*, originally a Roman army unit consisting of 300 to 600 legionaries), and they are studied *prospectively* in the sense that all the observations take place during the study according to a detailed protocol.

Some prognostic studies only comprise one cohort. One may, for instance, select a cohort of patients with a genetic abnormality (the cause) and then record the incidence of a particular disease (the effect) during the study period. This design, however, permits no comparisons and it would be much more informative to compare the observations in this cohort with those in a comparable cohort of persons without the genetic abnormality.

The randomized clinical trial is a special type of prospective cohort study where, in contrast to simple prognostic studies, the causal factor is introduced by active intervention and the patients are allocated at random to ensure that the two cohorts are comparable. This type of research, which represents the gold standard for testing new treatments, was discussed in detail in Chapter 6.

The *case-control study* also serves to analyse causal relationships, but the procedure is very different. Two groups of people are selected: the cases and the controls. The cases are characterized by presenting the effect in question, typically a particular disease, and the controls are characterized by the absence of this effect, typically normal people. The frequency of the assumed causal factor is recorded in both groups. A paediatrician who wishes to investigate

Table 8.1 Cohort and case-control studies. If the data represent the results of a comparative cohort study, the table is read horizontally. We calculate a/(a + b) and c/(c + d), i.e. the probability that members of the two cohorts develop the effect. If the data represent the results of a case-control study, the table is read vertically. We calculate a/(a + c) and b/(b + d), i.e. the probability that cases and controls presented the alleged causal factor.

		Effect		
		+	−	
Cause	+	a	b	a + b
	−	c	d	c + d
		a + c	b + d	

the relationship between splenectomy after abdominal trauma and the later development of pneumococcal sepsis might record the frequency of a history of splenectomy in a sample of children with pneumococcal sepsis (the cases) and then compare this frequency with that in a comparable group of children without pneumococcal sepsis (the controls). The detection of a difference between these frequencies would suggest a causal relationship, but it would not tell him anything about the magnitude of the risk of developing a sepsis after splenectomy. This type of case-control study is sometimes labelled retrospective as it incorporates information (the history of splenectomy) that was recorded before the start of the study. Other case-control studies are conducted within a carefully planned cohort study where the information has been gathered prospectively. Because the terms prospective and retrospective studies can be confusing they should be avoided.[217]

The difference between cohort studies and case-control studies is illustrated by Table 8.1, which shows that the two designs require different calculations. The results of cohort studies are often analysed by determining the relative risk, RR, which is the ratio between P(effect|cause) in the two groups. It is calculated as follows:

$$RR = \frac{a/(a + b)}{c/(c + d)}$$

Case-control studies do not permit such 'horizontal' calculations in the fourfold table as the number of cases and the number of controls were decided upon by the researcher. Instead the odds ratio, OR, is calculated, according to this formula:

$$OR = \frac{a/c}{b/d} = \frac{ad}{bc}$$

The odds ratio serves as a good approximation to the relative risk if the frequency of the effect is small, i.e. $a \ll (a + b)$ and $c \ll (c + d)$. A relative risk or an odds ratio of one means that the researchers did not find an association.

Assets and limitations of cohort studies

There are good possibilities of ensuring that the collected data are reliable in studies where future data collection is planned in accordance with a detailed protocol, but they are laborious and expensive if the cohorts are large and the observation period long. It is also important to distinguish between randomized and non-randomized cohort studies as the former are far more reliable (see Chapter 6).

Randomized trials can sometimes be difficult or impossible to perform. If we wished to compare the effects of breastfeeding with the effects of formula feeding, it might be hard to find a sufficient number of women in Europe who would be willing to be randomized to the two intervention groups. Most mothers would of course already have decided to breastfeed their baby. It might therefore be necessary to accept that the mothers, and not a randomization procedure, decided which type of milk to use. In this case, the results must be interpreted very cautiously. We must assume that breastfeeding mothers also differ in other respects from those mothers that do not breastfeed their babies, and such differences could very well be the cause of any differences between the children in the two groups. In Africa it was less clear what was best for the baby if the mother had been infected with human immunodeficiency virus (HIV). Breastfeeding increases the risk of HIV transmission from the mother whereas formula feeding increases the risk of diarrhoea if the mother has to use polluted water as a solvent. Several randomized trials have been carried out in such settings.[218]

The non-randomized cohort studies are a type of observational studies where a group of people are followed over time, and if treatments are instituted or stopped, this is part of usual clinical practice. Such studies are more reliable than case-control studies and they permit the demonstration of several effects of one cause, but the demonstration of a statistical association between two factors does not necessarily imply that the association is causal. One must always consider other interpretations, cf. the vaccination example on p. 55 that illustrated that it may sometimes be difficult to distinguish between real causes, common causes and concomitant causal factors. Confounding of that kind is only excluded in unbiased randomized trials.

Non-randomized cohort studies may provide an alternative to randomized trials when they, for some reason, cannot be carried out, and they can be useful supplements to randomized trials, as these are often too small or too short-term to identify rare or slowly developing harms. They may also elucidate benefits and harms of new treatments when they have become routine and are used by less well-educated clinicians and in types of patients that were not recruited for the carefully controlled randomized trials, e.g. elderly patients with several diseases and treatments. Finally, non-randomized studies can serve to generate interesting hypotheses that can be tested in randomized trials.

Assets and limitations of case-control studies

In many cases, case-control studies are much easier to do than cohort studies. In the example above, two cohorts of people with and without a genetic abnormality were followed to find out how many in each group developed a certain disease, but in that case it would have been much easier to study the occurrence of the genetic abnormality in groups of people with and without the disease.

Case-control studies may be used to demonstrate several causes of one effect but this type of research is often problematic, partly because the quality of the studies is often low, and partly because the results can be difficult to interpret.[219] It requires considerable attention and expertise on the part of the reader of journal articles to identify the possible sources of error, some of which deserve special mention.

Case-control studies, just like other scientific studies, require meticulous planning. It is necessary to write a protocol that states the hypotheses to be tested, the necessary definitions, and the in- and exclusion criteria for choosing the cases and the controls. As noted above, case-control studies are sometimes performed within the framework of a cohort study where the necessary data are registered continuously in accordance with the protocol. Thus, in large randomized trials, case-control studies can be conducted to reveal the possible causes of rare outcomes that may be related to factors other than the studied treatments. Sometimes, however, no such detailed protocol is prepared[220] and for that reason alone the results of the study may be difficult to interpret.

It is particularly important to choose a relevant control group and to ensure that the cases and the controls are sufficiently comparable, but that is not always easy. In studies aimed at determining the causes of a particular disease it may be useful to compare patients with the disease with patients suspected of the disease. For instance, women with a tumour in a breast who had their suspicion of breast cancer confirmed by microscopy may be compared with similar women who had normal breast tissue in their tumour. However, even this procedure is not safe. Malignant and benign breast lesions may have some causal factors in common and the study may therefore produce false negative results.

It is always difficult to reconstruct what happened in the past, and case-control studies that collect information retrospectively are much more unreliable and sensitive to confounding than prospectively planned cohort studies. The note in an old hospital record that some patient was subjected to a splenectomy is undoubtedly true, but the information that a patient suffered from pneumonia, rheumatoid arthritis or diarrhoea, or that he presented a duodenal ulcer at endoscopy, is much less reliable, as the diagnostic criteria used in the daily routine are rarely very precise. In most cases registers of diagnoses and causes of death are also unreliable[221] and they should not be used for research purposes unless they have been validated.

Information about past events is particularly unreliable when it depends on the memory of the participants in the study. If, for instance, a group of patients with ulcerative colitis and a group of healthy persons are asked whether or not they have ever suffered from eczema, it is only to be expected that the patients, who are more interested in the possible causes of the disease than the controls, will search their memory more thoroughly. Such recall bias may easily lead to a difference between the recorded rates of eczema in the two groups.

The interview technique may also be a source of bias. If, for instance, the group of cases is interviewed before the group of controls, the interviews of the controls may be less thorough than those of the cases, because the interviewer grew tired, or they may be more thorough, because the interviewer gradually improved his technique. Preferably, cases and controls should be interviewed in random order, but that is very rarely done.

Blinding is also an important principle that could be used more often in case-control studies. The interviewer need not know which of the interviewees are cases and which are controls, and, by including irrelevant questions in the questionnaires, both interviewers and patients may be kept ignorant of the hypotheses to be tested.

The medical literature illustrates only too well the importance of these and many other methodological problems, as there is no limit to causal associations that have been 'proved' by case-control studies. A series of studies, for instance, suggested a connection between a history of induced abortion and the development of breast cancer, and a much-quoted meta-analysis concluded that the risk increase was 30% (corresponding to an odds ratio of 1.3 with 95% confidence interval 1.2 to 1.4).[222] A Swedish team, however, found no association (odds ratio 0.95) and, when they consulted a register recording all abortions and corrected the information provided by the women, they even found that abortion had a protective effect, the risk of cancer being reduced by 37% (odds ratio 0.63).[223] Probably recall bias played an important role in the first study, as the women with breast cancer may have been more willing than the controls to admit that they had had an abortion.

Later, a large cohort study, including 1.5 million women, conclusively exploded these myths, as it was found that the relative risk was 1.00 (95% confidence interval 0.94 to 1.06).[224] A recent meta-analysis also failed to demonstrate an association overall, but the risk was significantly increased in 'retrospective studies' and significantly decreased in 'prospective studies'.[225]

Treatment of menopausal women with hormone replacement therapy also shows how misleading the results of non-randomized studies can be. As noted previously (p. 125), it was predicted that the hormones would decrease the risk of heart disease as they had a favourable effect on certain blood lipids. This view was supported by several cohort and case-control studies and a meta-analysis showed that the risk of developing heart disease was decreased by 50%.[226] Thereafter, the hormones were used by millions of women, partly with the justification that they protected against heart disease. Later, a large randomized trial showed, surprisingly, that hormones increase the risk of heart disease.[154] It should be noted that the meta-analysis was not done well as it did not take account of the fact that women who choose hormones have a higher socioeconomic status than other women, but even after adjustment for this confounder the risk for heart disease was not increased.[227]

As these examples illustrate, case-control studies often give rise to false benefits and false harms, and some experienced epidemiologists therefore use a rule of thumb not to be impressed by alleged harms demonstrated in non-randomized studies unless the risk is increased by at least a factor of three, corresponding to a risk increase of 200%.[228] It is also necessary to look at the confidence interval, as even an odds ratio of 20 is not too convincing if the number of people is so small that the confidence interval ranges from 2.2 to 114.

It follows that non-randomized studies should not be used to evaluate the possible beneficial effects of our treatments, as in most cases the expected effect is much smaller than the magnitude of bias that often occurs in such studies.[229]

Other designs

Cross-sectional studies are often the easiest ones to do. Data from one or more groups of people are collected at one moment in time, and associations in the data are analysed by means of appropriate statistical tests. It may, however, be difficult to establish what is the cause and what is the effect, as illustrated by the difficulties of determining the relationship between Helicobacter pylori infection and the development of duodenal ulcers, or that between unemployment and alcoholism (p. 56). In other cases, only one interpretation is possible. If, for example, an association is found between a certain tissue type and the occurrence of rheumatoid arthritis, it is, of course, the tissue type which predisposes to arthritis and not the arthritis which changes the tissue type.

One should also watch out for longitudinal interpretations of cross-sectional data. Once a textbook provided the information that the prevalence of intermittent claudication was 1.4% in 40–49-year-old men and 7.0% in 70–79-year-olds. In women, the corresponding figures were 1.9% and 1.0%. A longitudinal interpretation of these data, taken at face value, would mean that throughout life more and more men developed the disease, whereas more and more women were cured. It was, however, not a cohort study where the same people had been observed for 30 years, but two sets of cross-sectional data from different populations, and the high incidence among younger women probably reflected that during this period more young women had adopted the habit of smoking.

It has also been shown in cross-sectional studies that the frequency of Helicobacter infection of the stomach is correlated to age (in such a way that approximately 30% of 30-year-old men and 60% of 60-years-olds are infected and so forth), and a longitudinal interpretation would suggest that throughout their lives more and more people get infected. Most people, however, are infected when they are quite young, and the association between the prevalence and the age reflects that for many years the risk of infection has decreased.

Cross-sectional studies are also associated with other sources of error. Once it was found that gallstones were diagnosed more frequently in duodenal ulcer patients than in patients without abdominal complaints. Did that mean that gallstones predisposed to duodenal ulcers or that duodenal ulcers predisposed to gall stones? Probably, neither of these explanations was true. The ulcer patients who sought medical advice because of their abdominal pain were frequently examined for gallstones before the ulcer diagnosis was made, and sometimes the investigation led to the demonstration of stones that caused no symptoms at all.

Similarly, it was once reported in a study of hospital patients that the rate of previous admissions to psychiatric institutions was higher among ulcer patients than in the background population, and it was suggested that psychological factors played a causal role in the development of this disease. However, it is also possible that duodenal ulcer patients with a psychiatric history were more liable to reach the hospital threshold than duodenal ulcer patients with no psychiatric problems. Such misinterpretation of hospital data is known as *Berkson's fallacy*.[230]

This presentation of different designs is by no means exhaustive. Hybrids exist, especially the *historical cohort study*. A surgeon, for instance, may wish to study his successes and failures with a particular surgical operation. He goes through the hospital notes at his unit from the past few years and, assuming that the patients were seen routinely in the out-patient department for a period of time, he records the results of the operation. This is a *retrospective* study in the sense that the data collection took place before the start of the study, but it is also a *cohort study*, as the surgeon follows a cohort of patients to see the results of his operation. This design shares the strength of other cohort studies that it permits the calculation of P(effect|cause), but it also shares the weakness of other retrospective studies that the data quality may be poor. The indications for doing the operation were not defined in advance and stated in a detailed protocol with in- and exclusion criteria, and probably the notes in the patients' records about the clinical status after the operation were quite unstructured. Therefore, the scientific value of such studies is very doubtful, but the results may be of some use for the purpose of quality control.

Descriptive statistics

The attitude of doctors towards statistics ranges from distrust to blind faith. Some dismiss statistical calculations as superfluous, arguing that a signal that is not sufficiently strong to be recognized without statistical hocus-pocus must be uninteresting, whereas others accept any result as long as it is supported by a P-value below 5%. This spectrum of attitudes probably reflects that the teaching of statistics in many medical schools is either too limited or too theoretical. Some years ago a survey among Danish doctors revealed that the majority did not know the correct interpretation of such basic concepts as a P-value, a standard deviation (SD) and a standard error (SE)[20], and probably the situation is much the same elsewhere.

The simplest form of statistics is concerned with the description and presentation of the data. The researcher cannot publish all his observations but

Table 8.2 Data from 19 patients with hyperthyroidism. The patients have been listed according to their serum thyroxin concentration.

Age (years)	Ophthalmopathy (+ or −)	Severity of symptoms (Dr NN's clinical index)	Serum thyroxin (nmol/L)		
59	−	8	126		
35	−	23	127		
51	+	14	131		
62	−	7	137	lower	
43	−	23	146 ← quartile		⎤
62	+	8	155		⎮
32	−	20	157		⎮
40	−	16	167		⎮
44	+	10	171		inter-
58	−	28	175 ← median		quartile
54	+	9	179		range
38	−	27	185		⎮
76	−	14	218		⎮
36	−	22	243	upper	⎮
55	−	34	250 ← quartile		⎦
43	+	25	256		
50	+	33	269		
22	−	35	333		
27	+	29	397		

must process and condense the results in such a way that as little information as possible is lost. He may, for instance, have studied a sample of 19 patients with hyperthyroidism and instead of publishing all the crude data shown in Table 8.2, he will make brief statements of the following kind:

Ophthalmopathy was found in 37% of the patients. This trivial statement shows that data processing always entails some loss of information. If the statement is read out of context, we cannot know if the experience is based on only 19 or on many more patients. The example also shows that the method of data processing depends on the level of measurement of the original data. The presence or absence of ophthalmopathy constitutes a binary scale, and a series of observations on that level are conventionally condensed to a *rate* in per cent.

The mean age of the patients was 46.7 years (SD 13.7). The age of a patient is recorded on an interval scale, and the researcher condensed the 19 observations by calculating the mean and the standard deviation (SD).

The calculation and interpretation of the standard deviation was explained earlier (p. 20), and Fig. 2.1 illustrated that the interval, delimited by the mean ± two standard deviations, encompasses approximately 95% of the observations provided that the distribution is Gaussian. Therefore, if this requirement is fulfilled, the reader may expect that the age of almost all patients in this small sample ranged from 19 to 74 years. Table 8.2 shows that this is not far from the truth as the youngest patient was 22 and the oldest 76 years. In other words the standard deviation serves to visualize the distribution of the original data. There is, however, one problem: biological distributions are rarely Gaussian and the reader who interprets the standard deviation in this way may be seriously misled.

The median concentration of serum thyroxine was 175 nmol/L and the inter-quartile range was 146 to 250 nmol/L. The concentration of thyroxine was also recorded on an interval scale, but the author chose not to calculate the mean and standard deviation. Instead he ranked the data, as shown in Table 8.2, and determined the quartiles by dividing the sample into four equal parts. The three quartiles are called the lower quartile, the median (or half-way value) and the upper quartile, and the range between the lower to the upper quartile is denoted the inter-quartile range.

The quartiles are special cases of *quantiles.* If the ranked results are divided up into 10 groups, the nine values at which the divisions occur are called *deciles,* and if a sufficiently large number of results are divided up into 100 groups the divisions are called *percentiles.* Sometimes other quantiles are used. When discussing the calculation of the normal range (p. 28) it was suggested that the highest and the lowest fortieth (or 2.5%) of the results were removed, the remaining observations constituting the observed 95% range. The inter-quartile range (for small samples) and the observed 95% range (for large samples) are better measures of the dispersion of the results than the total range, which may be influenced by a single, atypically extreme value. It is often necessary to perform interpolations when quantiles are determined; thus the median of 10 results (in ranking order) must be calculated as the average of the 5th and the 6th result.

The measurements of the serum thyroxine concentrations constitute an interval scale and, therefore, the author might have quoted the mean rather than the median concentration, but it would have been quite misleading to quote the standard deviation, as the distribution is not Gaussian; it is positively skew and resembles the distribution shown in Fig. 2.3a. Calculation of mean ± two standard deviations gives the result 201 ± 148 nmol/L, suggesting that almost all observations lay within the interval 53 to 349 nmol/L, which, as seen in Table 8.2, was not the case.

Doctor NN's clinical index was used to measure the severity of the patients' symptoms. The median score was 22, the total range 7 to 35, and the inter-quartile range 10 to 28. This statement is analogous to the previous one, and if the reader ranks the scores in Table 8.2, he will find that the statement is correct. A clinical index constitutes an ordinal scale as it must be taken for granted that the symptoms of a patient with a high score are more severe than those of a patient with a lower score, but it cannot be assumed that the relationship is linear and that the index also constitutes an interval scale. Therefore, it would have made little sense to calculate the mean, which requires an interval scale, and the standard deviation, which requires both an interval scale and a Gaussian distribution. This mistake is often found in medical papers.

These examples illustrate that the researcher condenses the original observations by the calculation of so-called *statistics*, and the choice of statistic depends on the level of measurement of the data. The minimum requirements are the following:

Statistic	Level of measurement
Rate	Nominal scale
Median and quantiles	Ordinal scale
Mean	Interval scale
Standard deviation	Interval scale and Gaussian distribution

It is, of course, always possible to reduce the level of measurement. In one of the examples the researcher reduced the interval measurements of thyroxine in nmol/L to an ordinal scale by ranking, determining the median and the quartiles, and he could have reduced the level of measurement even further to a binary (nominal) scale by distinguishing only between high, and normal or low, concentrations. It is not permissible, however, to increase the level of measurement, which he would have done if he had calculated the mean and the standard deviation of the clinical index.

Estimation

The rate of ophthalmopathy was 37% (95% confidence interval: 16% to 62%. Table 8.2 shows that 7 of the 19 patients suffered from ophthalmopathy, which means that the observed rate was 37%. The clinician, however, also wanted to estimate the 'true' rate, and for that purpose he calculated the 95% confidence interval. In statistical terminology the observed rate, which refers to the sample in question, is an example of a *statistic*, whereas the unknown 'true' rate, which refers to the underlying population, is an example of a *population parameter*. Therefore, the calculation of a confidence interval is also called *interval estimation of a parameter*. I introduce this terminology, as the use of such expressions is one of the major stumbling blocks when doctors wish to study textbooks on biostatistics.

The principle of estimation or calculation of confidence intervals was explained on p. 101, and here I shall only recapitulate briefly that in the long run we may expect to be right 19 out of 20 times, when we conclude that the population parameter (the 'true' rate) lies within the calculated interval. It was also emphasized, however, that this does not necessarily mean that we may be 95% confident that the true value lies within the interval in the individual case. We must take into account all available evidence about the problem in question. Perhaps the rate of opthalmopathy was much lower in other studies of similar patients, and perhaps our study was one of the rare cases where the confidence interval did not catch the true value.

The mean age of the 19 patients was 46.7 years (SE 3.1). This statement resembles the descriptive statement, mean and SD discussed above, but the meaning is very different. SE or SEM is the standard error of the mean, and it is calculated by means of this very simple formula where N is the number of patients:

$$SE = SD/\sqrt{N}$$

The standard error is of some interest to readers of medical papers as it permits them to calculate the confidence interval for the mean. For practical purposes the 95% confidence interval of the 'true' mean is sample mean $\pm$ 2 SE, and in this case this interval is 40.5 to 52.9 years.

In many cases the SE is quoted when the reader is not the least interested in knowing the true average, but wishes to assess the dispersion of the results, as in this example where the age distribution describes the included patients. It is the standard deviation, not the standard error, which serves that purpose, but of course it is quite easy to calculate two SD, if SE is known:

$$2SD = 2SE \times /\sqrt{N}$$

It follows, as mentioned above, that 95% of the patients had an age between 19 and 75 years.

The mean thyroxine concentration was 201 nmol/L (SE 17). This statement is analogous to the previous one, but there is a problem. The standard error cannot be used to calculate the confidence interval if the sample is small and if the distribution is markedly non-Gaussian. In this case the sample only comprised 19 patients and the distribution was skew to the right and, consequently, the reader cannot be very confident that the true mean lies within the interval 201 ± 34 nmol/L. It can, however, be shown that the Gaussian assumption is less important if the sample is large, and the calculation might have been considered sufficiently reliable, if the sample size had been, say, 100 patients. In our example it would have been better to calculate the median and the confidence interval of the median, which requires computer assistance.

The resting pressure of the lower oesophageal sphincter in 25 healthy people was 19 ± 3.0 mmHg (mean ± SE). Statements like this one are quite frequent in medical journals and the critical reader ought to realize at once that they are meaningless. The author only reported the value of one SE and it is easy to calculate that mean ± 2 SD = 19 ± 30 mmHg, which suggests that some of these people had a negative resting pressure. Obviously, the distribution was truncated and skew to the right as shown in Fig. 2.3e, p. 28. Therefore, SD cannot be used to describe the distribution of the observations, and, as the sample was small, SE cannot be used to calculate the confidence interval.

Expressions of the type *mean ± a* are common, and sometimes the author forgets to tell the reader what *a* means, i.e. whether it is one SE, two SE, one SD or two SD. The same problem occurs in histograms and graphs where the 'uncertainty' of the results is indicated by a vertical line, but where the author forgot to tell the reader what the line means.

Confidence intervals may be calculated for many other statistics, e.g. the difference between two rates (p. 133), the difference between two means, relative risks and odds ratios.

Testing hypotheses

Both cohort studies and case-control studies are examples of hypothetico-deductive research: The scientist:

1. Evolves a hypothesis as regards a possible cause–effect relationship;

2. Plans and carries out a suitable trial or survey; and

3. Tests to what extent the results of his trial or survey are compatible with the initial hypothesis. Some researchers, however, do not adhere to this plan.

Pseudohypothetico-deductive logic

Imagine a person who is looking out of the window at a large car park that is divided up into two parking areas, one of which is better sheltered than the other. He notices the make, the size and the colour of the different cars, and suddenly he discovers that there are many more red cars in the sheltered area (11 out of 50) than in the other (2 out of 48). He then does the appropriate statistical test (Fisher's exact test) finds that P = 0.01 and concludes, rather hastily, that owners of red cars prefer to park in a sheltered place. This is obviously a case of muddled thinking, but it is necessary to be able to pinpoint the flaw in the argument. The 'scientist' reversed the order of the first two steps of the sequence mentioned above. Presumably, he had no hypothesis in mind when he started to look at the cars. He more or less consciously noticed the distribution of Fords, Volvos, blue cars, black cars etc., and he only decided to do a significance test when he saw that the red cars were unevenly distributed. We are, both in our daily lives and in our research, witnesses to innumerable chance events, 5% of which are 'statistically significant' on the 5% level, 1% on the 1% level and so forth, and those who disregard this simple fact are prone to make hasty conclusions. The surprising fact is that many researchers indulge in this kind of *pseudohypothetico-deductive logic*. They make numerous observations and whenever they see something unusual they do a significance test and conclude that they have discovered a new regularity in Nature.

I referred to this kind of logic when I warned against 'fishing expeditions' on p. 136, but it also appears in other disguises. Different types of multiple regression analyses have become very popular, but sometimes the results are interpreted rather uncritically. Perhaps numerous data are recorded when patients enter a prognostic cohort study, and then it is tempting to analyse afterwards, by means of a regression analysis, which of these characteristics were significantly correlated to the patients' prognosis. That, however, amounts to no more than a sophisticated 'fishing expedition', if it was not clearly stated in the protocol which hypotheses were to be tested. The results of multiple significance testing should, of course, not be ignored, but their main purpose is the provision of ideas for future studies.

There are surprisingly many significant P-values in the medical literature[231] and it is clear that most of them are misleading.[231,232]

Wrong sampling unit

Clinical research is done on groups (samples) of patients and the sampling unit in the statistical analysis is one patient. In Table 4.2 (on p. 66), for instance, there were 111 patients. If we had discovered, when reading the original paper more carefully, that in fact it only comprised 70 patients, 41 of whom had been examined twice, the calculation of diagnostic rates would have made no sense. In that case the sample unit would not have been one patient, but one ultrasound examination, and the observations would no longer have been mutually independent; one would have expected the second examination in most of the 41 cases to give the same result as the first examination.

The same holds true of randomized trials. If a trial report describes 600 epileptic fits we take it for granted that we are dealing with 600 different patients. If some patients had contributed with more than one attack, the statistical calculations would have made no sense. One would have expected that many of those patients who tried the treatment several times would have responded the same way each time.

These examples may sound rather trivial, but nevertheless this fallacy, which is called the wrong sampling unit, often appears in medical papers in different disguises. One may, for instance, encounter the vascular surgeon who examined 150 patients, of whom 80 had unilateral and 70 bilateral arterial insufficiency. He thought that the 'sample' consisted of 220 diseased legs and based his statistical calculations on that figure. That is of course wrong, as two legs from the same person are not mutually independent. If one leg is under the influence of the patient's diabetes, so is the other. Probably, the most extreme example is the randomized trial of 58 patients, where the unit used for the statistical analysis was not a patient, but a joint. Altogether 3,944 joints had been examined, and the resulting P-value was 0.00000001 (or as it was stated in the paper, with far too many decimals: 0.979126×10^{-8}). Obviously, the units were not mutually independent: if in one patient the treatment had an effect on one tender joint, it probably also had an effect on the others.

This error is also seen for data on harms where a table may list the individual harms, e.g. number of patients with headache, dizziness and fractures, in each group. It would be meaningless to compare the total number of harms in the two groups with a statistical test as the same patient could have more than one harm, e.g. dizziness could lead to a fall and a fracture. Furthermore, such a procedure also overlooks the fact that some harms are more serious than others.

Epidemiologists make similar mistakes. In population surveys the effect of preventive measures is often related to the number of person-years, e.g. the sum of the number of years each person was treated. This method was once used in a study of malaria prophylaxis in Tanzania,[233] and it was overlooked that the risk of infection of a diplomat living in Dar es Salaam for one year is not the same as that of 26 tourists spending a fortnight in a rural area under primitive conditions. The same criticism may be raised against studies of the effect of contraceptive measures where the measure of effect is number of pregnancies per year.

Finally, I should mention cross-over trials (p. 122), where, for example, 50 patients receive two treatments in succession. Here it is not permissible to compare the 50 observations during treatment A with the 50 observations during treatment B, as these 100 observations are not mutually independent, but paired two by two. One must use special statistical tests (tests for paired observations) suited for this design, as mentioned below.

Sample size calculations

Authors of medical papers should indicate in the 'Methods' section how they determined the sample size. Sample size calculations require that the researchers, at the planning stage, make up their minds about the hypothesis to be tested and the statistical specifications of the trial. Readers of medical journals need not, of course, be able to do such calculations themselves, but they should know the general principles.

Assuming a binary measure of effect (e.g. cured/not cured), the researchers should, at the planning stage, consider the following three questions, the answers to which constitute the specifications of the trial:

1. What risk of committing a type I error are we willing to accept? This is the risk of concluding that the treatment effects differ when in fact they are identical, and the conventional answer is 5%. If, however, the new treatment is expensive and the disease not very serious, it might be more reasonable only to accept a type I error risk (significance level) of 1%, in order to minimize the risk of introducing the treatment if it is no better than the old one.

2. What therapeutic gain are we looking for? Obviously, the sample size would have to be very large, if the researcher was looking for a difference between treatment effects of 1%, whereas only a small trial would be needed to detect a therapeutic gain of 40% or more. Once again, the answer depends on the clinical problem. If it is a question of life or death, it is important not to overlook small therapeutic gains, and in that case a large trial is needed.

3. What risk of committing a type II error are we willing to accept. We may have decided when we answered question 2 that we were looking for a therapeutic

gain of, say, 10%, but we must realize that there is always the risk that we end up with a statistically non-significant result even when the difference between the treatment results is 10% or more. How large may that risk be? Many researchers accept type II error risks of 20% or more, which is surprising. If the disease is serious, one may well argue that the type II error risk ought to be smaller than the type I error risk, and in most cases they ought to be of the same order of magnitude.

If these questions have been answered, and if it is possible to predict roughly the effect rate in the control group, it is easy calculate the necessary number of patients, using the proper statistical formula[9,14] or a computer program.

Example: 'The trial was designed to have 80% power (with $\alpha = 0.05$*) to detect a difference between the cure rates of at least 10%, and the required sample size was 750 patients.'* This is a typical quote from the methods section of a report of a randomized trial. The answer to the first question, i.e. the significance level (which is often called α), was 5%, the answer to the second question was 10%, and the answer to the third question was 20% (the 'power' being 100% – type II error risk). The sample size calculation, using these specifications, showed that 750 patients were needed.

Interpretation of P-values

The sample size calculation, as described above, was done according to conventional statistical theory, but the reader of a medical paper who has to interpret the resulting P-values must adopt a wider perspective. This topic was discussed in Chapter 6 where it was pointed out that the reader's confidence in a P-value also depends on his confidence in the null hypothesis. I shall now illustrate this important point by means of a fictitious example.[234]

Imagine two clinical researchers, Dr Nobel and Dr Repeat. Dr Nobel aspired for the Nobel Prize, for which reason he evolved highly original (even far-fetched) hypotheses, which he then tested by suitable trials. Dr Repeat only repeated the research of others. He developed no original ideas, but whenever he read about a trial in an international journal that had given a significant result, he wanted to see if he could reproduce that finding.

First, we shall look at Dr Nobel's career as a researcher, and we shall assume (rather unrealistically) that he has done 1000 randomized clinical trials comparing two treatments. Further, we shall imagine that this series comprised 900 trials where the treatments were equal and 100 where one treatment was markedly better than the other. In real life, of course, we never know the truth,

Table 8.3 The research career of Dr Nobel.

		Truth		Total
		H_A	H_0	
Test result	$P \leq 0.05$	90	45	135
	$P > 0.05$	10	855	865
	Total	100	900	1000

but the assumption fits Dr Nobel's research strategy. He develops original ideas, and usually (9 out of 10 times) the idea is wrong.

We also make the assumption that Dr Nobel accepts the conventional significance level of 5% and that his samples of patients were always so large that the chance of overlooking a true difference was only 10%. In other words, this series of trials was characterized by a type I error risk of 5% and a type II error risk of 10%. These assumptions permit us to construct the fourfold table shown in Table 8.3.

H_0 (the null hypothesis) was true in 900 trials, but we must expect that Dr Nobel obtained a statistically significant result ($P \leq 0.05$), simply by chance, in 5%, i.e. in 45 of these trials. H_A (the alternative hypothesis) was true in 100 trials, but, considering the type II error risk, we must expect that Dr N obtained a statistically non-significant result ($P > 0.05$) in 10%, i.e. in 10 of these trials.

It then follows, as shown in Table 8.3, that Dr Nobel obtained a statistically significant result in 135 trials, and that in 33%, or 45, of these the null hypothesis was true. In other words, we can only be 67% confident that there is a difference between the treatments when Dr Nobel finds a statistically significant difference. We can, however, rely on his non-significant results as the null hypothesis was true in 855/865 = 99% of those cases where he found that $P > 0.05$.

We may analyse Dr Repeat's research career in exactly the same way. He had also done 1000 trials, but he had confined himself to repeating the research of others, and therefore it is reasonable to assume that most of those treatments that he compared had, in fact, different effects. For the sake of the numerical example, we shall say that the null hypothesis was true in only 100 trials and that the alternative hypothesis was true in 900 trials.

Assuming, as in the case of Dr Nobel, that the type I error risk is 5% and the type II error risk 10% we can illustrate Dr Repeat's career by means of Table 8.4. In 5% of the 100 trials where H_0 was true he obtained a statistically

Table 8.4 The research career of Dr Repeat.

		Truth		
		H_A	H_0	Total
Test result	$P \leq 0.05$	810	5	815
	$P > 0.05$	90	95	185
	Total	900	100	1000

significant result, and in 10% of the 900 trials where H_A was true he obtained a non-significant result.

It follows, as shown in the table, that Dr Repeat obtained a statistically significant result in 815 trials and that in 5 (i.e. in less than 1%) of these trials the null hypothesis was true. Therefore, the results of Dr Repeat must be interpreted very differently from those of Dr Nobel, as we can be more than 99% confident that there is a difference between the treatments when Dr Repeat finds a statistically significant difference. Dr Repeat's non-significant results, however, are not very informative as in those cases there is almost a 50% chance that the alternative hypothesis is true.

In other words, the records of Dr Nobel and Dr Repeat are similar from the perspective of conventional statistical theory, as for both series of trials the type I error risk was 5% and the type II error risk 10%. Nevertheless, the records are very different from the point of view of the reader of their papers who wishes to make up his mind to which extent he can rely on their significant results.

These examples provide important clues to the interpretation of P-values from the reader's point of view. Whenever we read the report of, for instance, a randomized clinical trial, we must consider whether the study belongs to Dr Nobel's or Dr Repeat's universe. If our prior confidence in the null hypothesis is high, due to theoretical considerations or the results of others, we may decide that the study belongs to Dr Nobel's universe and we shall not believe too much in a statistically significant P-value. If, on the other hand, we have good reasons to believe that the two treatments have different effects, we may refer the study to Dr Repeat's universe, and decide that, probably, the treatment is effective even when the P-value is, for instance, 0.10.

This approach can also be used to illustrate the importance of the sample size. Usually, it is taken for granted that the interpretation of the P-value has nothing to do with the size of the study, but it is easy to show that, other things being equal, one should have less confidence in a significant P-value if

Table 8.5 The research career of Dr Nobel if he had used fewer patients in his trials.

		Truth		
		H_A	H_0	
Test result	$P \leq 0.05$	25	45	70
	$P > 0.05$	75	855	930
	Total	100	900	1000

the study is small. The smaller the size of the sample, the greater the risk of committing a type II error, and if the two treatment groups are very small (e.g. 20 patients in each), the risk of obtaining a non-significant P-value may be 75% even when one treatment is considerably better than the other. Table 8.5 shows what would have happened, if Dr Nobel had done 1000 trials of that small size. As before, he would have committed a type I error (obtained a significant P-value) in 5% of those experiments where the null hypothesis was true, but now he would have obtained a non-significant result in perhaps 75% of those trials where the effects of the two treatments differed. He would only obtain a significant P-value in 25 of the 100 trials, where the alternative hypothesis was true. Consequently, he would obtain a significant P-value in 70 trials, and in 45 (64%) of these trials the null hypothesis would be true. In other words, if the sample size was that small, we should only be 36% confident that there was a difference between the treatment effects, when he obtained a statistically significant P-value.

Statistical tests

Readers of journal articles need some knowledge of the assumptions and interpretation of the most common significance tests. I shall mention some of those that are used to compare two groups of patients, and it will be seen that the choice of test depends on the scale of measurement of the observations.

Fisher's exact test (or possibly a chi-square-test) is used to compare two rates, i.e. observations on a *binary scale*. This would be the correct choice, if we wished to compare the rate of opthalmopathy in two groups of patients.

The two-sample rank sum test (Mann–Whitney U test) is used to compare two distributions of *ordinal scale* measurements. It would be the ideal test for comparing the distribution of Dr NN's clinical index in two samples.

The two-sample t-test (student t-test) is used to compare two distributions of interval scale measurements, on the assumption that the underlying distributions are approximately Gaussian and that they have the same standard deviation. The test is robust to violation of the Gaussian assumption if the sample is large, the standard deviations similar, and the distributions not too asymmetrical, but it must not be used if the sample is small and the distribution skew. Then the two-sample rank sum test is to be preferred.

Some tests are specially suited to the analysis of cross-over trials where the observations are paired, i.e. the sign test (or McNemar test), one-sample rank sum test (Wilcoxon test) and one-sample t-test. The assumptions are those already mentioned for the two-sample tests.

Examples

The following examples illustrate some problems frequently encountered in medical papers.

In a randomized trial, cure was reported in 15 of 23 patients receiving treatment A, and in 15 of 29 patients receiving treatment B (Fisher's exact test, P = 0.40). Thus, there was no difference between the effects of the two treatments. The choice of test was correct, but the conclusion wrong. The therapeutic gain was 65% − 52% = 13% and, if we calculate its 95% confidence interval[14] we will find that it is 13 ± 27%. Therefore, from a statistical point of view, it is possible that treatment A cured between 40% more patients and 14% fewer patients than treatment B.

42 patients with disease A and 21 patients with disease B were compared. The mean VLDL-concentration was 346 mg/L (SE 66 mg/L) in group A and 627 mg/L (SE 93 mg/L) in group B, the difference being statistically significant (P < 0.01, two-sample t-test). In this case the observations were measured on an interval scale, but it is easy to see that the Gaussian assumption was not fulfilled. In group B, SD = 93 × $\sqrt{21}$ = 426 mg/L and, consequently, the mean ± 2 SD is 627 ± 852 mg/L. This calculation suggests that some of the patients had a negative VLDL-concentration, which, of course, is impossible. The distribution was very skew and the sample small, so the two-sample rank sum test should have been used instead of the t-test. It might, however, have been permissible to use the t-test, if the sample had been much larger, e.g. 100 patients in each group.

Simvastatin treatment for 5½ years reduced the death rate from all causes by 30%. This is a quotation from a Danish Drug Directory (commonly used by doctors in that country), and it describes correctly the results of the Scandinavian Simvastatin Survival Study,[235] which was done to test the preventive effect of simvastatin in patients with ischaemic heart disease and hypercholesterolaemia. The relative risk of death comparing the treatment group and the control group was 0.71. This reduction of the death rate seems impressive, but the decision whether or not to use the treatment also depends on the absolute risk reduction, i.e. the therapeutic gain, and that information was not provided in the Directory. The original paper states that 11.5% of 2223 patients in the control group died, compared with 8.2% of 2221 patients in the treatment group. Therefore, the therapeutic gain was 3.3% (95% confidence interval: 2.4% to 4.2%). One might also have calculated NNT, i.e. the number of patients one needs to treat for $5^{1}/_{2}$ years in order to avoid one death, which in this case is 1/0.033 = 30 (p. 135). That kind of information is needed to assess, among other things, the economical consequences of introducing the treatment. It has been shown that the presentation of the results of clinical studies influences the reader's assessment of the efficiency of a treatment.[236]

In a large trial (almost 4000 patients), comparing clofibrate and placebo in patients at risk of myocardial infarction, the death rates in the two groups were almost identical (20.0% and 20.9%). However, a subgroup analysis revealed that the death rate was considerably reduced among those persons in the clofibrate group who had taken at least 80% of the prescribed medicine.[237] This result suggested that clofibrate had an effect after all. Further analysis, however, revealed that this conclusion was too hasty, as the death rate was reduced to the same extent among those persons in the control group who had taken at least 80% of their inactive tablets. Despite numerous attempts it was not possible to find differences in cardiovascular risk factors between those who took most of the medicine and those who did not that could explain the better survival. The example illustrates the danger of subgroup analyses. The results of this trial only suggest that those who comply with the requirements of the protocol fare better than those who do not, regardless of the content of the tablets.

Treatment A and treatment B were compared in a randomized clinical trial. A comparison of the patients' condition before treatment and after treatment revealed that those who received treatment A presented a significant improvement (one-sample rank sum test, P < 0.05) whereas those who received treatment B did not improve significantly (NS). The author of this paper asked the question whether the condition, in each treatment group, improved during the treatment period, and it is correct to use the one-sample rank sum test to answer this question, but the question is irrelevant. He did the trial to find out whether one treatment was better than the other, but these tests do not compare the treatment results. It is quite possible that the improvement in group A was just statistically significant (e.g. P = 0.04) and in group B just statistically non-significant (e.g. P = 0.06), and such a difference may easily arise by chance. Instead the treatment results in the two groups should have been compared by means of a two-sample test. The example also shows that it is always best to state the exact P-value, and the expression NS (non-significant) should never be used.

Forty-two (58%) of 73 patients who received treatment A were cured compared with 33 (43%) of 76 patients who received treatment B. Treatment A was found to be significantly more effective than treatment B (one-tailed chi-square test, P = 0.04). This example illustrates a problem that I have not yet mentioned. On p. 131 the P-value was defined as the probability of obtaining, by chance, a difference between the treatment results which numerically is as large as (or larger than) the one observed in the study. In this case the therapeutic gain was 58% – 43% = 15%, and, consequently, we expect the P-value to tell us the probability of obtaining a difference of at least 15%, either in favour of treatment A or in favour of treatment B, if the null hypothesis is true. This conventional P-value, which does not take into account the direction of the difference, is said to be two-sided or two-tailed. In this case, however, the author calculated the one-tailed P-value which is the probability of obtaining a difference of 15% or more in favour of treatment A, i.e. he ignored the possibility that treatment A might be less effective than B. From a practical point of view there is no problem. The reader should just multiply the P-value by two. In this case the conventional two-tailed P is 0.08, and the difference was statistically non-significant. Sometimes authors use one-tailed tests (halve their P-values) without mentioning that they have done so and that practice borders on fraud.

The company's worldwide database of trials was used to retrieve randomized trials of paroxetine for depression. Statements of this kind in industry-supported meta-analyses are not uncommon, and the reader should not accept the results. In this example, the authors had missed 12 trials that indisputably fulfilled the inclusion criteria for the meta-analysis.[238] It is only to be expected that trials performed by the manufacturer of a drug are more positive than similar trials performed by competing companies or by independent researchers. Trials performed by the companies are often biased by design, analysis or reporting.[161,210]

Correlation analysis

Medical papers also report other types of statistical analyses. They may contain diagrams like Fig. 8.1b, which shows the correlation between the serum

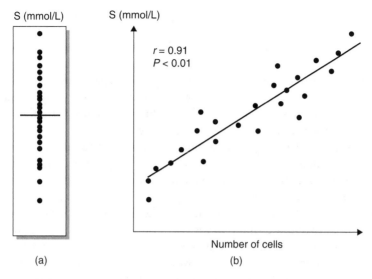

Fig. 8.1 a) The serum concentration of substance S in 25 patients. b) The correlation between the serum concentration of S and the number of a particular kind of cell in biopsy specimens from the same patients.

concentration of a substance S in 25 people and the number of cells of a particular type in tissue specimens from the same people. It is seen that the correlation is positive, as those patients who have a high content of S also tend to possess a large number of the cells in question. Usually a straight line, the regression line, is shown in such a diagram, and often the value of r, the correlation coefficient, and a P-value are quoted. It is the purpose of this presentation to explain the interpretation of these terms.

The researcher who did this study suspected that S was produced by a certain type of cell; he had noticed that the concentration of S varied from patient to patient (Fig. 8.1a), and he wanted to find out to what extent this variation could be explained by the fact that some patients possessed more cells of that particular type than others.

The favoured statistical measure of the dispersion of a series of observations is the variation around the mean, or $\sum(d^2)$, where, in this case, d is the difference between the concentration of S in the individual patient and the mean concentration of S in the whole sample. Therefore, in principle, the researcher measured the vertical distances between the individual points and the mean in Fig. 8.1a, squared these distances and calculated the sum. In correlation analysis this sum is called the *total variation* (or simply the sum of squares).

Next, as shown in Fig. 8.1b, the researcher related the concentrations of S to the number of cells in each patient, and, in order to interpret that relationship, he once again determined the variation of S, only this time he calculated the variation round the regression line, i.e. in principle, he measured the vertical distances between the points and the line, squared those distances and calculated the sum. This sum is called the *residual variation*. The regression line has been constructed in such a way that the residual variation around that line is smaller than the variation around any other line.

It is seen at a glance that the residual variation (the variation around the line) is much smaller than the total variation (the variation around the mean), which means that part of the variation in the concentration of S is explained by the variation in the number of cells in the patients in question. The explained variation is the difference between the total and the residual variation.

The meaning of this terminology is grasped most easily by considering two extremes, perfect correlation and no correlation at all. If the correlation had been perfect, all the points in Fig. 8.1b would have been situated on the regression line, and the residual variation would have been zero, meaning that the total variation had been fully explained. If, on the other hand, there had been no correlation, the points would have been evenly scattered, and the regression line would have been horizontal (on the level of the mean concentration of S). The residual variation would have been identical with the total variation, and nothing would have been explained.

The *correlation coefficient, r*, or the *determination coefficient, r^2*, are used to indicate the strength of the correlation. Usually, r is quoted, but r^2 is easier to interpret, as shown by this formula:

$$r^2 = \frac{\text{explained variation}}{\text{total variation}}$$

In our example, $r = 0.91$ and consequently $r^2 = 0.83$. This means that the explained variation is 83% of the total variation, i.e. that 83% of the variation in the concentration of S is explained by the fact that some patients have more cells of the particular type than others. The residual variation is only 17% of the total variation around the mean in Fig. 8.1a. The word 'explained' in these examples must of course not be taken at face value, as a positive or negative correlation between the y- and x-values does not necessarily imply that the variation of y is caused by the variation of x. It is also possible that the variation of x is caused by that of y or that both variations have a common cause.

In this example, the correlation was positive, and r was positive. The correlation may also be negative (the larger the value of x, the smaller the value of y), and in that case r would be negative. Thus the correlation coefficient varies from −1 (perfect negative correlation) over 0 (no correlation) to 1 (perfect positive correlation).

The correlation coefficient is a numerical characteristic of that particular sample, and as such it is subject to random variation. It may be larger or smaller than the 'true' correlation coefficient of the population, and, therefore, it is necessary to consider the possibility that the truth is that there is no correlation at all. This possibility is tested by a special significance test. In the example $r = 0.91$ and P < 0.01, which means that there is less than a 1% chance of obtaining an r value which differs that much from zero, if in fact there is no correlation at all. It is also possible to calculate the 95% confidence intervals of r and r^2.

Conventional correlation analysis assumes that the measurements have been recorded on an interval scale and that both the x-values and the y-values form a Gaussian distribution. If these assumptions are not fulfilled, it is necessary to use a ranking method, such as a *Spearman test*, and to calculate a rank correlation coefficient (R_S), which is tested against zero just like the conventional correlation coefficient. R_S and r are almost identical, if the distribution is Gaussian.

The following examples illustrate some of those hazards of correlation analyses that are sometimes ignored by clinical researchers.

A strong negative correlation was found between the gastric acid production and the age in a sample of 250 men with duodenal ulcer (P < 0.0001). These authors mistakenly believed that the correlation is strong when the P-value is small. In this case, $r = -0.56$ and $r^2 = 0.31$ which means that the correlation was quite weak. Only 31% of the variation in acid production is explained by the age variation. However, the author had studied so many patients that it is extremely unlikely that this weak correlation was a chance finding.

The clinical index in 80 patients and the collagen content of their liver biopsies showed a significant positive correlation (r = 0.28 and P = 0.01). The data and the regression line are shown in Fig. 8.2. The assumptions of the analysis, however, were violated as the distributions of both variables were far from Gaussian and, in addition, the clinical index is not measured on an interval scale, but on an ordinal scale. In this case, the authors ought to have done a Spearman test, which would have revealed that the P-value was 0.20.

Fig. 8.3 shows the correlation between the serum concentrations of two substances, Y and X. A Spearman test gave the result $R_S = 0.71$, P < 0.001. In this case the choice of test presented no problem, but in spite of that the analysis made little sense. The text shows that we are not dealing with one sample of 38 people, but with two samples: 17 normal controls and 21 patients suffering

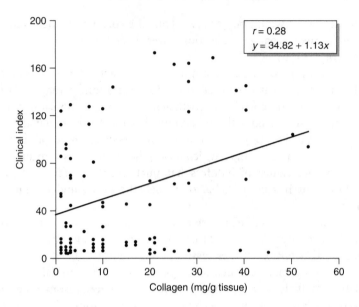

Fig. 8.2   The correlation between a clinical index and the collagen content of biopsies from 80 patients with a particular disease.

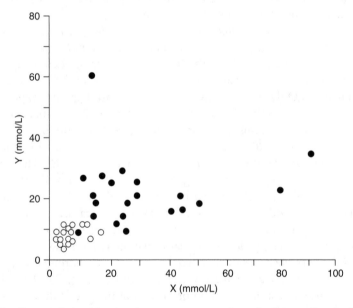

Fig. 8.3   The correlation between the serum concentrations of substance X and substance Y in 17 healthy people (open circle) and 21 patients with a particular disease (black circle).

from a particular disease. If we look at each of these samples in isolation, there is no obvious correlation between X and Y. The positive correlation only appears when we combine the samples, and that is impermissible. This is sometimes called the 'mouse–elephant' phenomenon. Probably, there is no positive correlation between the age and length of adult mice, nor between the age and length of adult elephants, but if we analysed a combined sample of 50 mice and 50 elephants, we should obtain a highly significant positive correlation and a minute P-value. There would be 50 points in the lower left corner and 50 in the upper right corner of the coordinate system.

Life table analysis

512 patients with a particular type of leukaemia were allocated at random to treatment A or treatment B. The Kaplan–Maier plots (Fig. 8.4) show that the patients receiving treatment A fared better than those receiving treatment B (logrank test:

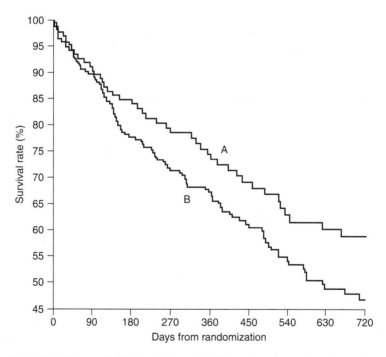

Fig. 8.4 Life table graph (Kaplan–Maier plot) illustrating the results of a randomized clinical trial.

P = 0.02). The cumulative two-year survival rate was 58% in group A and 46% in group B. Each 'step' on the graphs, which are often called Kaplan–Maier plots, represents the death of one patient, and they illustrate well the results of this trial. The simplicity of the illustration, however, is somewhat deceptive. The reader of this paper might notice that the trial ran from 1 January 1996 to 30 June 1998, during which period all patients fulfilling the entry criteria were admitted and seen regularly. On the latter date the trial closed, and no more observations were made. Consequently, those patients who were admitted within the last year of the trial period were observed for less than two years. How then is it possible to calculate the two-year survival rate?

This type of analysis is very useful and therefore I shall explain the basic principles.[9,239,240] Imagine a small prognostic study which aims at estimating the one-year survival rate of patients suffering from a particular disease. The trial period was 18 months (1 January 1997 to 30 June 1998) and during that period of time seven patients with this disease were seen. The crude observations are shown in Table 8.6a. It is seen that the first patient was

Table 8.6 Life table from a small prognostic study with seven patients. a) Date of entry, date of exit and status at exit. b) Day of entry for all patients has been labelled day 1 and the patients have been listed according to the length of the observation time.

Patient No.	Date of entry	Date of exit	Status at exit
a)			
1	19.01.04	30.06.05	Still alive
2	20.01.04	01.10.04	Died
3	12.05.04	16.02.05	Died
4	24.06.04	03.10.04	Died
5	12.10.04	30.06.05	Still alive
6	19.12.04	30.06.05	Still alive
7	05.01.05	31.05.05	Died
b)			
4	1	101	Died
7	1	146	Died
6	1	193	Still alive
2	1	255	Died
5	1	261	Still alive
3	1	280	Died
1	1	528	Still alive

observed for more than one year before the closing date (30 June 1998). The fifth and the sixth patients were also alive on the closing date, but had been observed for less than one year. The remaining four patients died during the study. In Table 8.6b this information has been reorganized. The day of entry for all patients has been called day 1 and the patients have been ranked according to the observation time. Now we may regard this sample as a small cohort of patients who all entered the study on the same day, but were observed for varying periods of time until they died or until the closure of the trial.

The statistician then calculates the survival rate whenever one of the patients leaves the cohort. On day 101 one patient died which means that the survival rate that day was 6/7 or 0.86. On day 146 one of the remaining six patients died, meaning that the survival rate that day was $5/6 = 0.83$. On day 193 one of the remaining five patients was lost to the cohort, but he was still alive so the survival rate on that day was one. Now only four patients were left, and, consequently, the survival rate on day 255 when one of them died was only $3/4 = 0.75$. On day 261 one of the remaining three patients was lost to follow-up, leaving two, which means that the survival rate on day 280 when one patient died was only 50%. The last patient survived until the trial closed.

Next, the statistician calculates the successive cumulative survival rates. The chance that a patient entering the trial on day one will survive day 101 and 146 is $0.86 \times 0.83 = 0.71$, the chance that he will survive also day 255 is $0.86 \times 0.83 \times 0.75 = 0.53$, and the chance that he will also survive also day 280 is $0.87 \times 0.83 \times 0.75 \times 0.50 = 0.27$. This is the cumulative one-year survival time. Fig. 8.5 is a Kaplan–Maier plot which, just like Fig. 8.4, shows the successive reduction of the cumulative survival rate.

Patients No. 5 and 6 illustrate well the advantage of these rather cumbersome calculations, which are usually done by a computer. They were not observed for a full year, but they are included in the calculation until the time when they left the cohort. The cumulative one-year survival rate incorporates the information that they survived that long. In large studies there are many such patients, and their inclusion may greatly influence the end result.

It is possible to calculate the 95% confidence interval of the cumulative survival rate, and it is also possible to compare the survival of two cohorts by means of a special significance test, the so-called logrank test. This was done in the example illustrated by Fig. 8.4. It is important to note that the test does not just compare the cumulative survival rates, but the differences throughout the whole course of the study.

The readers need to know how many patients were still being followed up at various times since they entered the study to judge the reliability of the study,

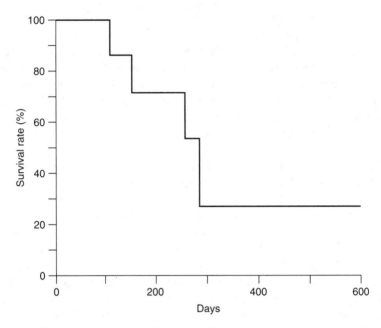

Fig. 8.5 Life table graph (Kaplan–Maier plot) illustrating the results of a small single-cohort prognostic study.

and this information should be given below the survival curve. In a recent observational study of 484 patients with screening-detected lung cancer the authors had reported a rather narrow confidence interval for 10-year survival after the diagnosis, although very few patients had been followed up for more than five years (despite still being alive) and only two people remained in the study after 10 years.[241] Such information is not reliable. We should also remember that observational studies of survival of patients with screening-detected cancer are highly unreliable because of overdiagnosis of harmless cases.[242]

Life table analysis is not only used in survival studies. It is also extremely useful for the analysis of other types of events, such as recurrences of a disease (e.g. recurrent myocardial infarctions), the development of complications (e.g. cerebrovascular attacks in cohorts of hypertensive persons) or the development of metastases in patients with malignant diseases.

References

Those references marked with an asterisk are particularly useful for further studies.

*1. Faber, K. *Nosography in Modern Internal Medicine*. London: Humphrey Milford, 1923.

*2. Sackett, D.L., Richardson, W.S., Rosenberg, W. *et al*. *Evidence-Based Medicine*. New York: Churchill Livingstone, 1997.

*3. Feinstein, A.R. *Clinical Judgment*. Baltimore: Williams & Wilkins, 1967.

4. Lusted, L.B. *Introduction to Medical Decision Making*. Springfield: C.C. Thomas, 1968.

5. Galen, R.S., and Gambino, R.S. *Beyond Mormality: The Predictive Value and Efficiency of Medical Diagnoses*. New York: Wiley, 1975.

*6. Murphy, E.A. *The Logic of Medicine*. Baltimore: Johns Hopkins University Press, 1976.

*7. Feinstein, A.R. *Clinical Biostatistics*. Saint Louis: Mosby, 1977.

8. Weinstein, M.C and Fineberg, H.V. *Clinical Decision Analysis*. Philadelphia: Saunders, 1980.

*9. Pocock, S.J. *Clinical Trials: A Practical Approach*. Chichester: John Wiley & Sons, Ltd, 1983.

*10. Feinstein, A.R. *Clinical Epidemiology: The Architecture of Clinical Research*. Philadelphia: W.B. Saunders Company, 1985.

*11. Feinstein, A.R. *Clinimetrics*. New Haven: Yale University Press, 1987.

*12. Andersen, B. *Methodological Errors in Medical Research*. Oxford: Blackwell Scientific, 1990.

*13. Wulff, H.R., Pedersen, S.A. and Rosenberg, R. *Philosophy of Medicine*. 2nd edition. Oxford: Blackwell Scientific, 1990.

*14. Altman, D.G. *Practical Statistics for Medical Research*. London: Chapman & Hall, 1991.

*15. Beauchamp, T.L. *Philosophical Ethics. An Introduction to Moral Philosophy*. 2nd edition. New York: McGraw-Hill, 1991.

*16. Sackett, D.L., Haynes, R.B., Guyatt, G.H. *et al. Clinical Epidemiology: A Basic Science for Clinical Medicine.* 2nd edition. Boston: Little, Brown and Company, 1991.

*17. BMA's Ethics Science and Information Division. *Medical Ethics Today: Its Practice and Philosophy.* London: BMJ Publishing Group, 1993.

18. Gillon, R. (ed). *Principles of Health Care Ethics.* Chichester: John Wiley & Sons, Ltd, 1993.

*19. Armitage, P. and Berry, G. *Statistical Methods in Medical Research.* 3rd edition. Oxford: Blackwell Science, 1994.

20. Wulff, H.R., Andersen, B., Brandenhoff, P. *et al.* What do doctors know about statistics? *Stat. Med.* 1987; **6**:3–10.

21. Lindley, D. *Making Decisions.* London: Wiley-Interscience, 1971.

22. Harpestreng, H. *Liber Herbarum* (13th century, in Latin and Danish). P. Hauberg, ed. Copenhagen: Hafnia, 1936.

23. Stevens, O. On the theory of scales of measurement. *Science* 1946; **103**: 677–80.

24. Huskisson, E.C. Measurement of pain. *Lancet* 1974; **2**:1127–31.

25. Gøtzsche, P.C. Sensitivity of effect variables in rheumatoid arthritis: a meta-analysis of 130 placebo controlled NSAID trials. *J. Clin. Epidemiol.* 1990; **43**: 1313–8.

26. Heart Failure Society of America. The Stages of Heart Failure: NYHA Classification [Web Page]. 2006; Available at http://www.abouthf.org/questions_stages.htm.

27. Apgar, V., Holiday, D.A., James, S. *et al.* Evaluation of the newborn infant. *JAMA* 1958; **168**:1985–8.

28. Knaus, W.A., Draper, E.A., Wagner, D.P. *et al.* APACHE II: a severity of disease classification system. *Crit. Care Med.* 1985; **13**:818–29.

29. Gøtzsche, P.C. Methodology and overt and hidden bias in reports of 196 double-blind trials of nonsteroidal, antiinflammatory drugs in rheumatoid arthritis. *Controlled Clin. Trials* 1989; **10**:31–56 (amendment:1989;10:356).

30. Thornley, B., Adams, C. Content and quality of 2000 controlled trials in schizophrenia over 50 years. *BMJ* 1998; **317**:1181–4.

31. Higgins, I. and Cochrane, A. Epidemiological studies of coronary disease. *Br. J. Prev. Soc. Med.* 1963; **17**:153–65.

32. Anonymous. Why did I ask for this pathological investigation? *Lancet* 1957; **ii**:890.

33. Hansen, U.M. [Oral measurement of body temperature. Clinical use of an electronic thermometer (Craftemp)]. *Ugeskr Laeger* 1991; **153**:3535–7.

34. Dodd, S.R., Lancaster, G.A., Craig, J.V. *et al.* In a systematic review, infrared ear thermometry for fever diagnosis in children finds poor sensitivity. *J. Clin. Epidemiol.* 2006; **59**:354–7.

35. Garland, L.H. Studies on the accuracy of diagnostic procedures. *Am. J. Roentgenol.* 1959; **82**:25–8.

36. Yerushalmy, J., Harkness, J.T., Cope, J.H. *et al.* The role of dual reading in mass radiography. *Am. Rev. Tub.* 1950; **61**:443–63.

37. Spitzer, R.L., Cohen, J., Fleiss, J.L. *et al.* Quantification of agreement in psychiatric diagnosis. A new approach. *Arch. Gen. Psychiatry* 1967; **17**:83–7.

38. Koran, L.M. The reliability of clinical methods, data and judgments. *N. Engl. J. Med.* 1975; **293**:642–6 & 695–701.

39. Herlev Hospital Study Group. Diagnostic decision-process in suspected pulmonary embolism. *Lancet* 1979; **1**:1336–8.

40. Feinstein, A.R. and Cicchetti, D.V. High agreement but low kappa: I. The problems of two paradoxes. *J. Clin. Epidemiol.* 1990; **43**:543–9.

41. Cicchetti, D.V. and Feinstein, A.R. High agreement but low kappa: II. Resolving the paradoxes. *J. Clin. Epidemiol.* 1990; **43**:551–8.

42. Feinstein, A.R. A bibliography of publications on observer variability. *J. Chronic Dis.* 1985; **38**:619–32.

43. Gjørup, T., Agner, E., Jensen, B.L. *et al.* The endoscopic diagnosis of gastric ulcer. A randomized clinical trial of interobserver variation and bias induced by knowledge of the radiological diagnosis. *Scand. J. Gastroenterol.* 1985; **20**:554–8.

44. Gjørup, T., Agner, E., Jensen, L.B. *et al.* The endoscopic diagnosis of duodenal ulcer disease. A randomized clinical trial of bias and of interobserver variation. *Scand. J. Gastroenterol.* 1986; **21**:261–7.

45. Gjørup, T., Bugge, P.M. and Jensen, A.M. Interobserver variation in assessment of respiratory signs. Physicians' guesses as to interobserver variation. *Acta Med. Scand.* 1984; **216**:61–6.

46. Gjørup, T., Bugge, P.M., Hendriksen, C. *et al.* A critical evaluation of the clinical diagnosis of anemia. *Am. J. Epidemiol.* 1986; **124**:657–65.

47. Frisch, T., Simonsen, L. and Hilden, J. [Observer variation and accuracy in the clinical diagnosis of ascites]. *Ugeskr Laeger* 1991; **153**:1864–8.

48. Korsgaard, B., Marcussen, H., Wulff, H.R. *et al.* [The expanded histamine test as a clinical aid]. *Ugeskr Laeger* 1968; **130**:1657–65.

∗49. Moynihan, R. and Cassels, A. *Selling Sickness: How the World's Biggest Pharmaceutical Companies are Turning Us All into Patients.* New York: Nation Books, 2005.

50. Horton, R. Lotronex and the FDA: a fatal erosion of integrity. *Lancet* 2001; **357**:1544–5.

∗51. Welch, H.G. *Should I Be Tested for Cancer? Maybe Not and Here's Why.* Berkeley: University of California Press, 2004.

52. Frankel, S., Smith, G.D., Donovan, J. *et al.* Screening for prostate cancer. *Lancet* 2003; **361**:1122–8.

53. Gøtzsche, P.C. and Nielsen, M. Screening for breast cancer with mammography. *Cochrane Database Syst. Rev.* 2006; (4):CD001877.

54. Raffle, A.E., Alden, B., Quinn, M. *et al.* Outcomes of screening to prevent cancer: analysis of cumulative incidence of cervical abnormality and modelling of cases and deaths prevented. *BMJ* 2003; **326**:901–4.

55. Brodersen, J. Measuring psychosocial consequences of false-positive screening results – breast cancer as an example. (PhD thesis). University of Copenhagen. Copenhagen: Månedsskrift for Praktisk Lægegerning (ISBN 87-88638-36-7), 2006.

56. Moynihan, R., Heath, I. and Henry, D. Selling sickness: the pharmaceutical industry and disease mongering. *BMJ* 2002; **324**:886–91.

57. Pilgaard, S., Krag, E. and Wulff, H.R. [Routine roentgen examination of the thorax and electrocardiography in a gastroenterological out-patient clinic. Useful or unnecessary examinations?] (English summary). *Ugeskr Laeger* 1975; **137**:2817–20.

58. Swedish Council on Technology Assessment in Health Care (SBU). *Preoperative Routines*. Stockholm: SBU, 1989.

59. Winkens, R.A., Pop, P., Grol, R.P. *et al.* Effects of routine individual feedback over nine years on general practitioners' requests for tests. *BMJ* 1996; **312**:490.

60. Riggs, B.L., Hodgson, S.F., O'Fallon, W.M. *et al.* Effect of fluoride treatment on the fracture rate in postmenopausal women with osteoporosis. *N. Engl. J. Med.* 1990; **322**:802–9.

61. Jones, F.A. (ed). *Richard Asher Talking Sense*. London: Pitman Medical, 1972.

62. Garrison, F.H. *An Introduction to the History of Medicine*. 4th edition. Philadelphia: Saunders, 1929.

63. Pedersen, S.A. Disease entities and open systems. In: Querido, A., van Es, L.A. and Mandema, E. (eds). *The Discipline of Medicine. Emerging Concepts and Their Impact on Medical Research and Medical Education*. Amsterdam: North Holland, 1984.

64. Goldberger, A.L. Non-linear dynamics for clinicians: chaos theory, fractals, and complexity at the bedside. *Lancet* 1996; **347**:1312–4.

65. Weiss, J.N., Garfinkel, A., Spano, M.L. *et al.* Chaos and chaos control in biology. *J. Clin. Invest.* 1994; **93**:1355–60.

*66. Nesse, R.M. and Williams, G.C. *Evolution and Healing. The New Science of Darwinian Medicine*. London: Phoenix, 1996.

67. McKeown, T. *The Origins of Human Disease*. Oxford: Basil Blackwell, 1988.

68. With, C. *Mavesaarets kliniske Former, dets Diagnose og Behandling* (in Danish). Copenhagen: Gyldendal, 1881.

69. Jennings, D. Perforated peptic ulcer. Changes in age-incidence and sex-distribution in the last 150 years. *Lancet* 1940; **i**:395–8 & 444–7.

70. Kendell, R.E. *The Role of Diagnosis in Psychiatry*. Oxford: Blackwell Scientific, 1975: 72.

71. Riis, P. and Anthonisen, P. The differential diagnosis between ulcerative colitis and Crohn's disease of the colon. In: Gregor, O., Riedl, O. (eds). *Modern Gastroenterology*. Stuttgart: Schattauer, 1969: 912.

72. Lipsky, P.E. Rheumatoid arthritis. In: Fauci, S.A., *et al.* (eds). *Harrison's Principles of Internal Medicine*. 14th edition. New York: McGraw-Hill, 1998: 1885.

73. Mackie, L.J. *The Cement of the Universe. A Study of Causation*. London: Oxford University Press, 1974.

74. Getz, L., Kirkengen, A.L., Hetlevik, I. *et al.* Ethical dilemmas arising from implementation of the European guidelines on cardiovascular disease prevention in clinical practice. *Scand. J. Prim. Health Care* 2004; **22**:202–8.

75. Zeta (pseudonym). *The Diagnosis of the Acute Abdomen in Rhyme.* London: H.K. Lewis, 1955.

76. Smidt, N., Rutjes, A.W., van der Windt, D.A. *et al.* Quality of reporting of diagnostic accuracy studies. *Radiology* 2005; **235**:347–53.

77. Puylaert, J.B., Rutgers, P.H., Lalisang, R.I. *et al.* A prospective study of ultrasonography in the diagnosis of appendicitis. *N. Engl. J. Med.* 1987; **317**:666–9.

78. Whiting, P., Harbord. R., Main, C. *et al.* Accuracy of magnetic resonance imaging for the diagnosis of multiple sclerosis: systematic review. *BMJ* 2006; **332**:875–84.

79. Johnsen, R., Bernersen, B., Straume, B. *et al.* Prevalences of endoscopic and histological findings in subjects with and without dyspepsia. *BMJ* 1991; **302**: 749–52.

80. Horvath, W.J. The effect of physician bias in medical diagnosis. *Behav. Sci.* 1964; **9**:334–40.

81. Grande, P., Christiansen, C., Pedersen, A. *et al.* [Rational diagnosis of acute myocardial infartion. Efficiency calculations]. *Ugeskr Laeger* 1980; **142**:1565–9.

82. Harvey, R.F. Indices of thyroid function in thyrotoxicosis. *Lancet* 1971; **2**:230–3.

83. Cobb, S. On the development of diagnostic criteria. *Arthritis Rheum.* 1960; **3**:91–5.

*84. STARD group. STARD Initiative (Standards for Reporting of Diagnostic Accuracy) [Web Page]. 2007; Available at http://www.consort-statement. org/stardstatement.htm.

85. Reid, M.C., Lachs, M.S. and Feinstein, A.R. Use of methodological standards in diagnostic test research: getting better but still not good. *JAMA* 1995; **274**:645–51.

86. Schmidt, L.M. and Gøtzsche, P.C. Of mites and men: reference bias in narrative review articles: a systematic review. *J. Fam. Pract.* 2005; **54**:334–8.

87. Schmidt, W.A., Kraft, H.E., Vorpahl, K. *et al.* Color duplex ultrasonography in the diagnosis of temporal arteritis. *N. Engl. J. Med.* 1997; **337**:1336–42.

88. Schonberg, M.A., McCarthy, E.P., Davis, R.B. *et al.* Breast cancer screening in women aged 80 and older: results from a national survey. *J. Am. Geriatr. Soc.* 2004; **52**:1688–95.

89. Meador, C.K. Non-disease: a problem of overdiagnosis. *Diagnostica (Ames Corp)* 1969; **3**:10–1.

90. Meador, C.K. The art and science of nondisease. *N. Engl. J. Med.* 1965; **272**:92–5.

91. Bull, J.P. The historical development of clinical therapeutic trials. *J. Chron. Dis.* 1959; **10**:218–48.

92. Gotfredsen, E. *Medicinens Historie (in Danish).* Copenhagen: Busck, 1950.

93. Major, R.H. *Classic Descriptions of Disease.* 3rd edition. Springfield: CC Thomas, 1945.

94. Lasagna, L. *The Doctor's Dilemmas.* London: Gollancz, 1962.

95. Clendening, L. *Source Book of Medical History.* New York: Dover, 1960.

96. Gavaret, J. *Principes généraux de statistique médicale* (quoted from Danish translation). Copenhagen: Reizel, 1840.
97. Fenger, C.E. Om den numeriske metode (in Danish). *Ugeskr Læger* 1839; 1:305–15 & 321–5.
98. Louis, P.C.A. *Recherches sur les effects de la saignée dans quelques maladies inflammatoires.* Paris: Bailleres, 1835.
99. Faber, K. Historical outline of medical therapy. In: Faber K. *Lectures on Internal Medicine.* New York: Hoeber, 1927.
100. Löwy, I. *The Polish School of Philosophy of Medicine.* Philosophy of medicine series, No. 39. Dordrect: Kluwer, 1990.
101. Bieganski, W. *Medizinische Logik* (translated from Polish). Würzburg: Curt Kaubitzsch, 1909.
102. Kaye, M.D., Rhodes, J., Beck, P. *et al.* A controlled trial of glycopyrronium and l-hyoscyamine in the long-term treatment of duodenal ulcer. *Gut* 1970; 11:559–66.
103. Anonymous. Anticholinergics and duodenal ulcer. *Lancet* 1970; 2:1173.
104. Sturdevant, R.A., Isenberg, J.I., Secrist, D. *et al.* Antacid and placebo produced similar pain relief in duodenal ulcer patients. *Gastroenterology* 1977; 72:1–5.
105. Peterson ,W.L., Sturdevant, R.A., Frankl, H.D. *et al.* Healing of duodenal ulcer with an antacid regimen. *N. Engl. J. Med.* 1977; 297:341–5.
106. Hróbjartsson, A., Gøtzsche, P.C. Is the placebo powerless? An analysis of clinical trials comparing placebo with no treatment. *N. Engl. J. Med.* 2001; 344:1594–602.
107. Hróbjartsson, A., Gøtzsche, P.C. Placebo interventions for all clinical conditions. *Cochrane Database Syst. Rev.* 2004; (3):CD003974.
108. Jacobsen. Belladonna mod kighoste (in Danish). *Bibliotek Læger* 1809; 1:105–6.
109. Williams, S.G. and Westaby, D. Management of variceal haemorrhage. *BMJ* 1994; 308:1213–7.
110. Bornman, P.C., Krige, J.E. and Terblanche, J. Management of oesophageal varices. *Lancet* 1994; 343:1079–84.
111. Sharara, A.I. and Rockey, D.C. Gastroesophageal variceal hemorrhage. *N. Engl. J. Med.* 2001; 345:669–81.
112. Gøtzsche, P.C. and Hróbjartsson, A. Somatostatin analogues for acute bleeding oesophageal varices. *Cochrane Database Syst. Rev.* 2005; (1):CD000193.
113. Galton, F. Regresssion towards mediocrity in hereditary stature. *J. Anthropol. Instit. Great Britain Ireland* 1885; 15:246–63.
114. Chalmers, I. and Matthews, R. What are the implications of optimism bias in clinical research? *Lancet* 2006; 367:449–50.
115. Grünbaum, A. The placebo concept in medicine and psychiatry. *Psychol. Med.* 1986; 16:19–38.
116. Brody, H. *Placebos and the Philosophy of Medicine.* Chicago: University of Chicago Press, 1980.
117. Gøtzsche, P.C. Is there logic in the placebo? *Lancet* 1994; 344:925–6.

118. Kienle, G.S. and Kiene, H. Placebo effect and placebo concept: a critical methodological and conceptual analysis of reports on the magnitude of the placebo effect. *Forschende Komplementärmedizin* 1996; **3**:121–8.

119. Beecher, H.K. The powerful placebo. *JAMA* 1955; **159**:1602–6.

120. Kleijnen, J., de Craen, A.J., van Everdingen, J. *et al.* Placebo effect in double-blind clinical trials: a review of interactions with medications. *Lancet* 1994; **344**:1347–9.

121. Thomas, K.B. General practice consultations: is there any point in being positive? *Br. Med. J.* 1987; **294**:1200–2.

122. Knipschild, P. and Arntz, A. Pain patients in a randomized trial did not show a significant effect of a positive consultation. *J. Clin. Epidemiol.* 2005; **58**: 708–13.

123. Hodnett, E.D., Gates, S., Hofmeyr, G.J. *et al.* Continuous support for women during childbirth. *Cochrane Database Syst. Rev.* 2003; (3):CD003766.

124. Kunz, R., Vist, G. and Oxman, A.D. Randomisation to protect against selection bias in healthcare trials. *Cochrane Database Methodol. Rev.* 2002; (4):MR000012.

125. Fibiger, J. Om serumbehandling af difteri. *Hospitalstidende* 1898; **6**:309–25 & 337–50.

126. Hróbjartsson, A., Gøtzsche, P.C. and Gluud, C. The controlled clinical trial turns 100 years: Fibiger's trial of serum treatment of diphtheria. *BMJ* 1998; **317**: 1243–5.

127. Medical Research Council. Streptomycin treatment of pulmonary tuberculosis. *BMJ* 1948; **272**:92–5.

128. Brynner, R.S.T. *Dark Remedy: The Impact of Thalidomide and its Revival as a Vital Medicine.* New York: Perseus Publishing, 2001.

129. Saunders, J. Alternative, complementary, holistic ... In: Greaves, D. and Upton H. (eds). *Philosophical Problems in Health Care.* Avebury: Avebury, 1996: 103–25.

130. Coulter, H.L. Homoeopathy. In: Salmon, J.W. (ed). *Alternative Medicines.* London: Tavistock, 1985.

131. Caplan, R.L. Chiropractic. In: Salmon, J.W. (ed). *Alternative Medicines.* London: Tavistock, 1985.

132. Meade, T., Dyer, S., Browne, W. *et al.* Low back pain of mechanical origin; randomised comparison of chiropractic and hospital outpatient treament. *BMJ* 1990; **300**:1431–7.

133. Assendelft, W.J., Morton, S.C., Yu, E.I. *et al.* Spinal manipulative therapy for low back pain. *Cochrane Database Syst. Rev.* 2004; (1):CD000447.

134. James Randi Educational Foundation. One Million Dollar Paranormal Challenge. 2006; Available at www.randi.org/research/index.html.

135. Ernst, E. Adulteration of Chinese herbal medicines with synthetic drugs: a systematic review. *J. Intern. Med.* 2002; **252**:107–13.

136. Mostefa-Kara, N., Arnaud, P., Pines, E. *et al.* Fatal hepatitis after herbal tea. *Lancet* 1992; **340**:674.

137. Popper, K.R. *Conjectures and Refutations*. 5th edition. London: Routledge and Kegan Paul, 1974.

138. King, M., Nazareth, I., Lampe, F. *et al.* Impact of participant and physician intervention preferences on randomized trials: a systematic review. *JAMA* 2005; **293**:1089–99.

139. Linde, K., Clausius, N., Ramirez, G. *et al.* Are the clinical effects of homeopathy placebo effects? A meta-analysis of placebo-controlled trials. *Lancet* 1997; **350**:834–43.

140. O'Dowd, A. New rules for homoepathic remedies anger UK peers. *BMJ* 2006; **333**:935.

∗141. *The Cochrane Library*. Chichester: Wiley, 2007.

142. Bernard, C.L. Introduction a l'étude de la médecine expérimentale, 1866, reprinted. London: Garnier-Flammarion, 1966.

∗143. CONSORT group. CONSORT statement (Consolidated Standards of Reporting Trials) [Web Page]. 2007; Available at http://www.consort-statement.org.

144. Van Spall, H.G., Toren, A., Kiss, A. *et al.* Eligibility criteria of randomized controlled trials published in high-impact general medical journals: a systematic sampling review. *JAMA* 2007; **297**:1233–40.

145. Jüni, P., Nartey, L., Reichenbach, S. *et al.* Risk of cardiovascular events and rofecoxib: cumulative meta-analysis. *Lancet* 2004; **364**:2021–9.

146. Jüni, P., Altman, D.G. and Egger, M. Systematic reviews in health care: Assessing the quality of controlled clinical trials. *BMJ* 2001; **323**:42–6.

147. Devereaux, P.J., Manns, B.J., Ghali, W.A. *et al.* Physician interpretations and textbook definitions of blinding terminology in randomized controlled trials. *JAMA* 2001; **285**:2000–3.

148. Haahr, M.T. and Hróbjartsson, A. Who is blinded in randomized clinical trials? A study of 200 trials and a survey of authors. *Clin. Trials* 2006; **3**:360–5.

149. Gøtzsche, P.C., Liberati, A., Torri, V. *et al.* Beware of surrogate outcome measures. *Int. J. Technol. Assess. Health Care* 1996; **12**:238–46.

150. Majeed, A.W., Troy, G., Nicholl, J.P. *et al.* Randomised, prospective, single-blind comparison of laparoscopic versus small-incision cholecystectomy. *Lancet* 1996; **347**:989–94.

∗151. Gøtzsche, P.C. Bias in double-blind trials (DrMedSci thesis). *Dan. Med. Bull.* 1990; **37**:329–36.

152. The Cardiac Arrhythmia Suppression Trial (CAST) Investigators. Preliminary report: effect of encainide and flecainide on mortality in a randomized trial of arrhythmia suppression after myocardial infarction. *N. Engl. J. Med.* 1989; **321**:406–12.

153. Moore, T.J. *Deadly Medicine*. New York: Simon and Schuster, 1995.

154. Rossouw, J.E., Anderson, G.L., Prentice, R.L. *et al.* Risks and benefits of estrogen plus progestin in healthy postmenopausal women: principal results from the Women's Health Initiative randomized controlled trial. *JAMA* 2002; **288**: 321–33.

155. Salpeter, S.R., Buckley, N.S., Ormiston, T.M. *et al.* Meta-analysis: effect of long-acting beta-agonists on severe asthma exacerbations and asthma-related deaths. *Ann. Intern. Med.* 2006; **144**:904–12.

156. Ioannidis, J.P., Evans, S.J., Gøtzsche, P.C. *et al.* Better reporting of harms in randomized trials: an extension of the CONSORT statement. *Ann. Intern. Med.* 2004; **141**:781–8.

157. Gøtzsche, P.C. Musculoskeletal disorders. Non-steroidal anti-inflammatory drugs. *Clin. Evid.* 2005; (14):1498–505.

158. Montori, V.M., Devereaux, P.J., Adhikari, N.K. *et al.* Randomized trials stopped early for benefit: a systematic review. *JAMA* 2005; **294**:2203–9.

159. Moher, D., Schulz, K.F., Altman, D. *et al.* The CONSORT statement: revised recommendations for improving the quality of reports of parallel-group randomized tirals. *JAMA* 2001; **285**:1987–91.

160. Altman, D.G., Schulz, K.F., Moher, D. *et al.* The revised CONSORT statement for reporting randomized trials: explanation and elaboration. *Ann. Intern. Med.* 2001; **134**:663–94.

161. Melander, H., Ahlqvist-Rastad, J., Meijer, G. *et al.* Evidence b(i)ased medicine – selective reporting from studies sponsored by pharmaceutical industry: review of studies in new drug applications. *BMJ* 2003; **326**:1171–3.

162. Hollis, S., Campbell, F. What is meant by intention to treat analysis? Survey of published randomised controlled trials. *BMJ* 1999; **319**:670–4.

163. Wulff, H.R. Confidence limits in evaluating controlled therapeutic trials. *Lancet* 1973; **2**:969–70.

∗164. International Committee of Medical Journal Editors. Uniform requirements for manuscripts submitted to biomedical journals [Web Page]. 2007; Available at http://www.icmje.org.

165. Yusuf, S., Wittes, J., Probstfield, J. *et al.* Analysis and interpretation of treatment effects in subgroups of patients in randomized clinical trials. *JAMA* 1991; **266**:93–8.

166. ISIS-2 (second international study of infarct survival) Collaborative Group. Randomised trial of intravenous streptokinase, oral aspirin, both, or neither among 17 187 cases of suspected acute myocardial infarction: ISIS-2. *Lancet* 1988; **ii**:349–60.

167. Healy, D. and Cattell, D. Interface between authorship, industry and science in the domain of therapeutics. *Br. J. Psychiatry* 2003; **183**:22–7.

∗168. Kassirer, J.P. *On the Take: How Medicine's Complicity with Big Business Can Endanger Your Health.* Oxford: Oxford University Press, 2005.

169. Gøtzsche, P.C., Hróbjartsson, A., Johansen, H.K. *et al.* Ghost authorship in industry-initiated randomised trials. *PLoS Med* 2007; **4**:e19.

170. Scherer, R.W., Langenberg P. and von Elm, E. Full publication of results initially presented in abstracts. *Cochrane Database Methodol. Rev.* 2005; (2):MR000005.

171. Chalmers, I., Murray, E. and Keirse, M.J.N.C. *Effective Care in Pregnancy and Childbirth.* Oxford: Oxford University Press, 1989.

*172. Higgins, J.P.T. and Green, S. (eds). Cochrane Handbook for Systematic Reviews of Interventions 4.2.6 [updated Sept 2006].

*173. Egger, M., Smith, G.D. and Altman, D.G. (eds). *Systematic Reviews in Health Care: Meta-Analysis in Context.* London: BMJ Publishing Group, 2001.

174. Chan, A.W., Hróbjartsson, A., Haahr, M.T. *et al.* Empirical evidence for selective reporting of outcomes in randomized trials: comparison of protocols to published articles. *JAMA* 2004; **291**:2457–65.

175. Egger, M., Smith, G., Schneider, M. *et al.* Bias in meta-analysis detected by a simple, graphical test. *BMJ* 1997; **315**:629–34.

176. Konstam, M.A., Weir, M.R., Reicin, A. *et al.* Cardiovascular thrombotic events in controlled, clinical trials of rofecoxib. *Circulation* 2001; **104**:2280–8.

177. Gifford, R.H. and Feinstein, A.R. A critique of methodology in studies of anticoagulant therapy for acute myocardial infarction. *N. Engl. J. Med.* 1969; **280**:351–7.

178. Moher, D., Pham, B., Jones, A. *et al.* Does quality of reports of randomised trials affect estimates of intervention efficacy reported in meta-analyses? *Lancet* 1998; **352**:609–13.

179. Antman, E.M., Lau, J., Kupelnick, B. *et al.* A comparison of results of meta-analyses of randomized control trials and recommendations of clinical experts: treatments for myocardial infarction. *JAMA* 1992; **268**:240–8.

180. Aspinall, R.L. and Goodman, N.W. Denial of effective treatment and poor quality of clinical information in placebo controlled trials of ondansetron for postoperative nausea and vomiting: a review of published trials. *BMJ* 1995; **311**:844–6.

181. Fergusson, D., Glass, K.C., Hutton, B. *et al.* Randomized controlled trials of aprotinin in cardiac surgery: could clinical equipoise have stopped the bleeding? *Clin. Trials* 2005; **2**:218–29; discussion 229–32.

182. Berlin, J.A., Begg, C.B. and Louis, T.A. An assessment of publication bias using a sample of published clinical trials. *J. Am. Stat. Assoc.* 1989; **84**:381–92.

183. Gilbert, J.P., McPeek, B. and Mosteller, F. Progress in surgery and anesthesia: benefits and risks of innovative therapy. In: Bunker, J.P. (ed). *Costs, Risks, and Benefits of Surgery.* New York: Oxford University Press 1977; 124–69.

184. Colditz, G.A., Miller, J.N. and Mosteller, F. How study design affects outcomes in comparisons of therapy. I: Medical. *Stat. Med.* 1989; **8**:441–54.

185. Miller, J.N., Colditz, G.A. and Mosteller, F. How study design affects outcomes in comparisons of therapy. II: Surgical. *Stat. Med.* 1989; **8**:455–66.

186. ALLHAT investigators. Major outcomes in high-risk hypertensive patients randomized to angiotensin-converting enzyme inhibitor or calcium channel blocker vs diuretic: The Antihypertensive and Lipid-Lowering Treatment to Prevent Heart Attack Trial (ALLHAT). *JAMA* 2002; **288**:2981–97.

187. Lieberman, J.A., Stroup, T.S., McEvoy, J.P. *et al.* Effectiveness of antipsychotic drugs in patients with chronic schizophrenia. *N. Engl. J. Med.* 2005; **353**: 1209–23.

188. Jones, P.B., Barnes, T.R., Davies, L. *et al.* Randomized controlled trial of the effect on quality of life of second- vs first-generation antipsychotic drugs in

schizophrenia: Cost Utility of the Latest Antipsychotic Drugs in Schizophrenia Study (CUtLASS 1). *Arch. Gen. Psychiatry* 2006; **63**:1079–87.

*189. Angell, M. *The Truth About the Drug Companies: How They Deceive Us and What To Do About It.* New York: Random House, 2004.

*190. Goozner, M. *The $800 Million Pill: The Truth Behind the Cost of New Drugs.* Berkeley: University of California Press, 2005.

*191. Abramson, J. *Overdo$ed America: The Broken Promise of American Medicine.* New York: Harper Collins, 2004.

*192. Krimsky, S. *Science in the Private Interest: Has the Lure of Profits Corrupted Biomedical Research?* Maryland: Rowman & Littlefield, 2003.

*193. Avorn, J. *Powerful Medicines: The Benefits, Risks, and Costs of Prescription Drugs.* New York: Vintage Books, 2005.

194. Engel, G.L. Commentary. In: Odegaard, C.E. *Dear Doctor. A Personal Letter to a Physician.* Menlo Park: The Henry J. Kaiser Family Foundation, 1986: 157.

195. Ewing, A.C. *Ethics.* London: English University Press, 1953: vi.

196. Kübler-Ross, E. *On Death and Dying.* New York: Macmillan, 1969.

197. Lunde, I.M. Patienters egenvurdering. Et perspektivskift (DrMedSci thesis) (English summary). Copenhagen: FADL's forlag, 1990.

198. Frøjk, M. Kronisk nyresyg (PhD thesis) (in Danish). Odense: Odense University, 1992.

199. Denzin, N.K. and Lincoln, Y.S. (eds). *Handbook of Qualitative Research.* Thousand Oaks: Sage, 1994.

200. Kollemorten, I., Strandberg, C., Thomsen, B.M. *et al.* Ethical aspects of clinical decision-making. *J. Med. Ethics* 1981; **7**:67–9.

201. The Gospel according to St. Matthew 7;12.

202. Stanley, J.M. The Appleton Consensus: suggested international guidelines for decisions to forego medical treatment. *J. Med. Ethics* 1989; **15**:129–36.

203. Wulff, H.R. Against the four principles: a Nordic view. In: BMA's Ethics Science and Information Division. *Medical Ethics Today: Its Practice and Philosophy.* London: BMJ Publishing Group, 1993: 277–86.

204. Thomsen, O.Ø., Wulff, H.R., Martin, A. *et al.* What do gastroenterologists in Europe tell cancer patients? *Lancet* 1993; **341**:473–6.

205. Marcus, P.M., Bergstralh, E.J., Zweig, M.H. *et al.* Extended lung cancer incidence follow-up in the Mayo Lung Project and overdiagnosis. *J. Natl. Cancer Inst.* 2006; **98**:748–56.

206. Wulff, H.R. The inherent paternalism in clinical practice. *J. Med. Philos.* 1995; **20**:299–311.

207. Sheldon, T. Dutch argue that mental torment justifies euthanasia. *BMJ* 1994; **308**:431–2.

*208. World Medical Association. Declaration of Helsinki: Ethical Principles for Medical Research Involving Human Subjects [Web Page]. 2007; Available at http://www.wma.net/e/policy/b3.htm.

209. Gøtzsche, P.C., Hróbjartsson, A., Johansen, H.K. *et al.* Constraints on publication rights in industry-initiated clinical trials. *JAMA* 2006; **295**:1645–6.
210. Safer, D.J. Design and reporting modifications in industry-sponsored comparative psychopharmacology trials. *J. Nerv. Ment. Dis.* 2002; **190**:583–92.
211. Bekelman, J.E., Li, Y. and Gross, C.P. Scope and impact of financial conflicts of interest in biomedical research: a systematic review. *JAMA* 2003; **289**:454–65.
212. Als-Nielsen, B., Chen, W., Gluud, C. *et al.* Association of funding and conclusions in randomized drug trials: a reflection of treatment effect or adverse events? *JAMA* 2003; **290**:921–8.
213. Heiberg. Studier over den statistiske Undersøgelsesmetode som Hjælpemiddel ved terapeutiske Undersøgelser (in Danish). *Bibliotek for Læger* 1897; **7**:1–40.
*214. Greenhalgh, T. *How to Read a Paper: The Basics of Evidence Based Medicine.* London: BMJ Publishing Group, 1997.
*215. STROBE group. STROBE Statement (STrengthening the Reporting of OBservational studies in Epidemiology) [Web Page]. 2007; Available at http://www.strobe-statement.org.
*216. PRISMA group. Statement (Preferred Reporting Items for Systematic reviews and Meta-Analyses) [Web Page]. 2007; Website in preparation.
217. Vandenbroucke, J.P. Prospective or retrospective: what's in a name? *BMJ* 1991; **302**:249–50.
218. Mbori-Ngacha, D., Nduati, R., John, G. *et al.* Morbidity and mortality in breastfed and formula-fed infants of HIV-1-infected women: A randomized clinical trial. *JAMA* 2001; **286**:2413–20.
219. Pocock, S.J., Collier, T.J., Dandreo, K.J. *et al.* Issues in the reporting of epidemiological studies: a survey of recent practice. *BMJ* 2004; **329**:883–7.
220. Feinstein, A.R. and Horwitz, R.I. Double standards, scientific methods, and epidemiologic research. *N. Engl. J. Med.* 1982; **307**:1611–7.
221. Gjersøe, P., Andersen, S.E., Molbak, A.G. *et al.* [Reliability of death certificates. The reproducibility of the recorded causes of death in patients admitted to departments of internal medicine]. *Ugeskr Laeger* 1998; **160**:5030–4.
222. Brind, J., Chinchilli, V.M., Severs, W.B. *et al.* Induced abortion as an independent risk factor for breast cancer: a comprehensive review and meta-analysis. *J. Epidemiol. Community Health* 1996; **50**:481–96.
223. Lindefors-Harris, B.M., Eklund, G., Adami, H.O. *et al.* Response bias in a case-control study: analysis utilizing comparative data concerning legal abortions from two independent Swedish studies. *Am. J. Epidemiol.* 1991; **134**:1003–8.
224. Melbye, M., Wohlfahrt, J., Olsen, J.H. *et al.* Induced abortion and the risk of breast cancer. *N. Engl. J. Med.* 1997; **336**:81–5.
225. Beral, V., Bull, D., Doll, R. *et al.* Breast cancer and abortion: collaborative reanalysis of data from 53 epidemiological studies, including 83000 women with breast cancer from 16 countries. *Lancet* 2004; **363**:1007–16.

226. Stampfer, M.J. and Colditz, G.A. Estrogen replacement therapy and coronary heart disease: a quantitative assessment of the epidemiologic evidence. *Prev. Med.* 1991; **20**:47–63.

227. Humphrey, L.L., Chan, B.K. and Sox, H.C. Postmenopausal hormone replacement therapy and the primary prevention of cardiovascular disease. *Ann. Intern. Med.* 2002; **137**:273–84.

228. Taubes, G. Epidemiology faces its limits. *Science* 1995; **269**:164–9.

*229. Deeks, J.J., Dinnes, J., D'Amico, R. *et al.* Evaluating non-randomised intervention studies. *Health Technol. Assess.* 2003; **7**:1–173.

230. Berkson, J. Limitations of the application of fourfold table analysis to hospital data. *Biomet. Bull.* 1946; **2**:47–53.

231. Gøtzsche, P.C. Believability of relative risks and odds ratios in abstracts: cross sectional study. *BMJ* 2006; **333**:231–4.

232. Sterling, T.D. Publication decisions and their possible effects on inferences drawn from tests of significance - or vice versa. *Am. Stat. Assoc. J.* 1959; **54**:30–4.

233. McLarty, D.G., Webber, R.H., Jaatinen, M. *et al.* Chemoprophylaxis of malaria in non-immune residents in Dar es Salaam, Tanzania. *Lancet* 1984; **2**:656–9.

234. Wulff, H.R. Magic of p values. *Lancet* 1988; **1**:1398.

235. Scandinavian Simvastatin Survival Study Group. Randomised trial of cholesterol lowering in 4444 patients with coronary heart disease: the Scandinavian Simvastatin Survival Study (4S). *Lancet* 1994; **344**:1383–9.

236. Naylor, C.D., Chen, E. and Strauss, B. Measured enthusiasm: does the method of reporting trial results alter perceptions of therapeutic effectiveness? *Ann. Intern. Med.* 1992; **117**:916–21.

237. Coronary Drug Project Research Group. Influence of adherence to treatment and response of cholesterol on mortality in the coronary drug project. *N. Engl. J. Med.* 1980; **303**:1038–41.

238. Jørgensen, A.W., Hilden, J. and Gøtzsche, P.C. Cochrane reviews compared with industry supported meta-analyses and other meta-analyses of the same drugs: systematic review. *BMJ* 2006; **333**:782–5 (full report: doi:10.1136/bmj.38973.444699.0B Published 6 October 2006).

*239. Peto, R., Pike, M.C., Armitage, P. *et al.* Design and analysis of randomized clinical trials requiring prolonged observation of each patient. I. Introduction and design. *Br. J. Cancer* 1976; **34**:585–612.

*240. Peto, R., Pike, M.C., Armitage, P. *et al.* Design and analysis of randomized clinical trials requiring prolonged observation of each patient. II. Analysis and examples. *Br. J. Cancer* 1977; **35**:1–39.

241. Henschke, C.I., Yankelevitz, D.F., Libby, D.M. *et al.* Survival of patients with stage I lung cancer detected on CT screening. *N. Engl. J. Med.* 2006; **355**:1763–71.

242. Welch, H.G., Woloshin, S., Schwartz, L.M. et al. Overstating the evidence for lung cancer screening. The International Early Lung Cancer Action Program (I-ELCAP study). *Arch Intern Med* 2007; **167**:26 Nov (in press).

Index